Self-Medication

Self-Medication

The Proceedings of the Workshop on Self-Care, held at the Royal College of Physicians, London, on 8th and 9th January, 1979

Edited by
J. A. D. Anderson
Professor of Community Medicine,
Guy's Hospital Medical School,
London

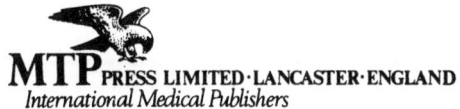
MTP PRESS LIMITED·LANCASTER·ENGLAND
International Medical Publishers

Published by

MTP Press Limited
Falcon House
Lancaster, England

ISBN 978-94-011-8145-7   ISBN 978-94-011-8143-3 (eBook)
DOI 10.1007/978-94-011-8143-3

Copyright © 1979 MTP Press Limited

Softcover reprint of the hardcover 1st edition 1979

British Libray Cataloguing in Publication Data

Workshop on Self-Care, Royal College of
    Physicians, 1979
    Self medication.
    1. Self medication — Great Britain —
    Congresses
    1. Title II. Anderson, John Allan Dalrymple
    615'.58   RM103

Typeset by Typecrafters Ltd., Preston
and printed by
Redwood Burn Ltd., Trowbridge & Esher

Contents

Contributors

J. A. D. Anderson
Department of Community Medicine
Guy's Hospital Medical School, London

J. M. Atkinson
Department of Community Medicine
University of Glasgow

P. N. Bennett
Royal United Hospital, Bath and
University of Bath

L. J. Christopher
Department of Clinical Pharmacology
and Therapeutics
Department of Geriatric Medicine
Royal Victoria Hospital, Dundee

J. Crooks
Department of Pharmacology
and Therapeutics
University of Dundee

S. Curry
Department of Pharmacology
and Therapeutics
The London Hospital Medical College

G. Cust
Health Education Council

J. Davis
National Consumer Council

J. Fry
General practitioner, Beckenham, Kent

G. R. Fryers
Proprietary Association of Great Britain

R. Goulding
Poisons Unit, Guy's Health District
London

A. J. Hedley
Department of Community Health
University of Nottingham

A. Herxheimer
Department of Pharmacology
Charing Cross Hospital Medical School,
London

J. G. Iles
General practice pharmacist

M. J. Linnett
Chairman of Council
Royal College of General Practitioners

J. McEwen
Department of Community Medicine
University of Nottingham

D. C. Morrell
General Practice Teaching and
Research Unit
St. Thomas's Hospital Medical School
London

7

SELF-MEDICATION

P. A. Parish
Department of Clinical and Social
Pharmacy, Welsh School of Pharmacy,
Cardiff

J. B. Spooner
Sterling Winthrop Group Limited
Surbiton, Surrey

T. G. Stewart
Department of Community Medicine
University of Glasgow

J. H. Walker
Department of Family and Community
Medicine,
University of Newcastle upon Tyne

J. P. Wells
Proprietary Association of Great Britain

Workshop Chairmen
The Lord Richardson
Chairman
Council for Postgraduate Medical Education
in England and Wales

N. J. B. Evans
Deputy Chief Medical Officer
Department of Health and Social Security

*Assistance with conference expenses and
preparation of this report was provided jointly by:
The Health Education Council and
The Proprietary Association of Great Britain.*

1

Historical background to self-care

J. A. D. ANDERSON

The discipline of community medicine can be regarded as the successor to public health and its practitioners, like the medical officers of health before them, should have a special interest in preventive medicine and the principals of positive health. Many members of the specialty receive formal postgraduate training in institutions dedicated to the goddess Hygeia whose powers were concerned particularly with maintaining health. It might seem more natural, therefore, that an opening chapter on self-care by a community physician should be devoted to some of the broader issues of the subject than are indicated by the subtitle of self-medication associated with this workshop. A puritanical diatribe on avoiding alcoholic and dietary excesses would have been seasonal, and that banker of health education, a homily on the dangers of smoking tobacco, would also have been appropriate — so too would exhortations to regulated exercise through recreation or by means of daily targets for such wholesome activities as jogging, ergonomic bicycling or press-ups.

All the above are highly relevant to any consideration of self-care in its broadest sense and attitudes on personal prevention and health maintenance may well have a limited place in the discussions associated with this conference. However, the main purpose of this Workshop is concerned with that aspect of self-care knows as self-medication; accordingly it is with the worship of Aesculapius rather than Hygeia that this introductory chapter is devoted, since it is to be hoped that consideration will only be given to the broader issues of self-care in the light of their relevance to that particular facet — self-medication — that forms the theme of this gathering.

In setting the scene it is usually helpful to have a working definition, and in the light of the views and opinions expressed in the precirculated papers (the substance of which forms Chapters 3 to 6) it would seem appropriate to suggest the following:

> The use for medicinal purposes of any substance for which therapeutic properties are claimed and which is packaged and sold to the public without medical prescription.

Since the dawn of history 'cures' for disease have developed along two parallel but often interwoven pathways [1]. These therapeutic approaches were originally based on the concept that human suffering arose from two different causes. On the one hand there were major diseases with a supernatural or religious basis which were seen as induced by the vengeance of an omnipotent being or god whose wrath had been provoked by deliberate or unintentional lapse, or who was seeking to test loyalties by the tribulation of disease. Such divine intervention could only be countered by spiritual therapy which would exorcise the demon responsible and expert advice, therefore, was essential. Depending on their inclinations and the sophistication of the community being served these expert healers were either priests or magicians.

The second curative pathway, also lost in the mists of time, was concerned with so-called simple remedies for minor ailments. Some may have been prehuman, as in the eating of grass by domestic pets; other appear to have arisen by the juxtaposition of *cause* and *cure* as in the case of stinging nettles and sorrel leaves. In any event the causative agent was obvious and the therapy familiar enough to be passed on to others without the intervention of a *qualified* healer.

As primitive scientists challenged the priesthood, and miasmata (from the moon or elsewhere) replaced spiritual deviance as the bases for major disease so successors to the priests and magicians developed into the orthodox practitioners and quacks of the middle ages. Technical advances in the use of alcohol, opium and other herbal remedies containing relatively potent drugs, together with a residuum of belief in magic, enabled the unscrupulous to lure the gullible away from reputable physicians and surgeons. This was no doubt made easier by the fact that much of the so-called orthodox advice of the day was ineffective and barbaric; indeed in the light of modern knowledge many of the practices were frankly dangerous.

The Medical Act of 1858 clarified the issue as to who could or could not practise medicine and most ethical apothecaries and leeches followed the physicians and surgeons of the Royal Colleges along the trail of respectability. Those who were excluded from the medical brotherhood had two courses open. On the one hand they could content themselves with being supplementary professionals with both their training and practising ethics determined largely by doctors — a state of affairs which has persisted for some into modern times. The alternative was to practise independently with all the allegations of quackery that such a course entailed. Those with neither training nor ethical standards joined the ranks of the exploiters and toured the country with one or more patent remedies.

Thus, in the nineteenth century sanctions against unqualified purveyors of healing potions were based on the issue of whether or not the practitioner was *licensed* rather than on the type of ingredients contained in the medications being dispensed. Indeed legislative control of home medicines has been a comparatively recent and much more drawn-out affair than the decisions inherent in the Medical Act of 1858. It is true that pharmacological ingredients have had to be specified and their quantities stated for a number of years. However, this information was not always obvious from a cursory glance at the package and even today the stated formula is likely to be unfamiliar to many lay purchasers. Furthermore, extravagant claims for therapeutic miracles persisted well into the twentieth century, though the restrictions have been gradually increased including an embargo on claims in the lay press about cures for such diseases as cirrhosis of the liver, duodenal ulcer, pernicious anaemia, psychoses, rheumatoid arthritis and tuberculosis. However, remedies for the relief of symptomatic ailments such as liverishness, acidity, bloodlessness, nervousness, rheumatism, or chronic cough were not forbidden and the distinction between these vague labels and the more specific ones was not necessarily clear in lay minds.

Any consideration of self-medication in modern Britain must take account of the introduction of a fully comprehensive National Health Service in 1948. Its predecessor of 1911 had provided for the care of a limited section of the population (mainly males of working age) and its terms of service included strong discouragements to expensive prescribing. The National Health Service proper extended the service to all sections of the community and is much more liberal in its prescribing regulations. Everyone now has direct access to primary care and it is clear that over 95% of the population are registered with a general practitioner [2]. Even those who are not registered, or who are temporarily removed from easy access to their own doctor and who wish to avail themselves of the service, may either consult an alternative general practitioner on a temporary basis or have direct access to hospital services through a casuality department.

The illogical conclusion to providing health services free at the point of consumption is that a stage may be reached where every trivial symptom becomes the topic of a professional consultation with no element of self-reliance by the public. On the other hand there can be no justification for self-medication which endangers health either because the ingredients are toxic in themselves, or because unscrupulous salesmanship suggests that potentially dangerous symptoms can be treated beneficially by inappropriate home medicines.

It would appear, therefore, that it is still possible to consider ailments under two broad headings: those which are serious and require the advice of medical practitioners or other experts, and those which are trivial or at least familiar to the individual. As far as the serious complaints are concerned there remains a need to decide which professions should be regarded as competent to advise on treatment; for the milder group safe home remedies are not only effective and safe if taken in appropriate dosage over a reasonable length of time but form an essential ingredient of the overall pattern of care if the health services are not to become inundated. Some authorities believed that the introduction of prescription charges might help in this respect but inflationary trends have resulted in the price of most medicaments exceeding the charges for even the simplest of home remedies.

Even if the balance between need and demand could be achieved in relation to prescribed medicines there would remain two important considerations in respect of self-medication. First the medicines must be safe; few dissent from this view, but what is safe for one person may be dangerous for another. I saw my first chloridine addict a hundred years after the passing of the Medical Act. She got one day's supply each week in the form of a prescription for 12 ounces of ipecac and morphine mixture dispensed as 'mist. expect. stim. double strength'; this she consumed as a single draught on the steps of the pharmacy and for the rest of the week she was self-reliant, purchasing an inordinate number of small bottles of tincture. Another supposedly safe home remedy, phenacitin, was consumed in considerable quantities until recently, and renal physicians are still caring for the late consequences of its open access. Such problems and the effects of reduced vigilance in the matter of prescribing supposedly controlled medicines such as dextroamphetamine and many hypnotics, originally believed to be non-addictive, has led to increasingly tight controls. Indeed there is currently a lobby to curtail self-medication still further by reducing the availability of home medicines and limiting their sale to registered pharmacies — presumably with the proviso that the pharmacist must be present at the time of sale in order to exert some sort of control.

The second point to be considered if self-medication is to have a natural place in the spectrum of care is that even safe home remedies become potentially dangerous if they are used mistakenly (or for too long) in the treatment of potentially serious diseases. There have been developments recently which should help the public in this respect. Thus the establishment of the Health Education Council should help to make people better informed about their health problems and assist them in the identification of potentially serious symptoms. The pharmaceutical industry also has accepted certain disciplinary standards in that members of the Proprietary Association of Great Britain have a vuluntary code of practice in respect of advertising and packaging. However, this should not lead to the assumption that all medical products available for self-care are necessarily covered by such criteria. For instance, the mail purchase of a seven-day supply of ginseng and vitamin E advertised as a 'health aid' in a widely circulated lay journal will bring with it copious literature which contains carefully worded indirect suggestions as to the therapeutic qualities of this extraordinary piece of polypharmacy. Today the claims are subdued in comparison with their counterparts of forty years ago since medicines, like any other commodity sold in the United Kingdom, must now conform to the provisions of the Trade Descriptions Act. Even so, there are likely to be a number of gullible readers who will believe that their exhaustion will be overcome and their sexual prowess enhanced by a full course of the treatment, to say nothing of the oblique hints that regular medication may bring about improvement in diabetes, heart desease, depression and insomnia.

Some aspects of the problems associated with self-medication have been explored by comparing those who attended a general practitioner with matched samples of those who had not done so for at least a year [3]. In common with many other studies [4, 5] it was found that around 63% overall had self-medicated within two weeks of the date of interview. The symptomatic history of the self-medication selected by the

Table 1.1 Evaluation of self-medication (symptoms treated by self-medication during the previous two weeks)

No. of subjects		Completely effective	Partially effective	Harmless	Harmful	Unclassifiable (panel disagreement)	Total symptom ≏ 100%
377	Attenders	98 (20.5%)	266 (53.3%)	53 (11.0%)	24 (5.0%)	40 (8.3%)	481
300	Non-attenders	102 (30.0%)	153 (45.0%)	38 (11.2%)	15 (4.4%)	32 (9.4%)	340
677	**Totals**	200 (24.4%)	419 (51.0%)	91 (11.1%)	39 (4.8%)	72 (8.8%)	821*

* 433 reported symptoms which were not treated have been omitted.

Table 1.2 Evaluation of self-medication (60 matched pairs with the same symptoms of similar severity)

	Completely effective	Partially effective	Harmless	Harmful	Unclassifiable	Total ≏ 100%
Attenders	2 (8.0%)	14 (64.0%)	4 (16.0%)	0 (0%)	5 (20%)	25
Non-attenders	10 (23.3%)	19 (44.2%)	4 (9.3%)	4 (9.3%)	6 (14.0%)	43
Totals	12 (17.9%)	33 (49.3%)	8 (12.0%)	4 (6.0%)	11 (16.4%)	68*

* 52 Patients who did not use self-treatment for their symptoms have been excluded.

two samples as stated to a lay interviewer were offered to a panel of three doctors. Where consensus was possible the panel took the view that 81% of self-medications were either completely effective or partially effective for the symptoms being treated (see Table 1.1). However, in 5% of the symptoms elicited (39 out of 821 symptoms presented by 677 people) it was suggested that the medication selected might be potentially harmful in the stated circumstances; there was, however, no significant difference in this respect between those who subsequently attended their doctors and those who did not.

Among the attenders it was noted that pain was often the stated cause for seeking medical advice. Since this pain factor and other indications of increasing severity are likely to have a bearing on whether or not a patient consults a doctor it was decided to study pairs of attenders and non-attenders who were further matched by the type and severity of their symptoms; 60 such pairs were identified and it was found that there were significantly more non-attenders than attenders who had indulged in self-midication during the two-week period under review (see Table 1.2). It was also noted that four of the self-medications used by 48 people with symptoms among the non-attenders were graded as potentially harmful; by way of contrast, none of the medications used by the 25 people with matching symptoms and who had treated themselves before attending the doctor were so graded. Studies were also made to try and identify psychosocial factors in which the attenders and non-attenders could be said to differ. There was a suggestion [6] that self-reliance by the non-attenders was greater than among the attenders, but the difference was not statistically significant — possibly because of the small numbers in the cohorts of matched pairs.

The chance of a potentially harmful outcome — even on the unsubstantiated criteria of this particular study — is likely to cause anxiety in relation to home medication and further research is obviously needed to explain the findings. It is unlikely that the active ingredients themselves in the quantities stipulated in a single dose would be considered harmful in the light of current medical knowledge. The question arises, therefore: are people self-medicating for too long because they are unaware of the inherent dangers?

In order to consider this possibility a second phase of the study looked at the appropriateness or otherwise of the management of the different symptoms including the speed with which patients attended their doctor (or failed to attend). On the basis of these criteria there were 20% of symptoms among non-attenders and 17% among attenders which were

Table 1.3 Appropriateness of self-care (based on the treatments used and the delay in seeking medical advice)

	Appropriate	Inappropriate	Total No. $\simeq 100\%$
Upper respiratory tract infections	14.6 (75.6%)	47 (24.4%)	193
Musculoskeletal	119 (88.1%)	16 (11.9%)	135
Gastrointestinal	201 (89.3%)	24 (10.7%)	225
Cardiovascular	75 (65.2%)	40 (37.8%)	115
Psychological disorders	66 (69.5%)	29 (30.5%)	95

deemed to have been handled inappropriately by the panel of doctors. Depending on the system to which the complaint related this inappropriateness ranged from 35% of symptoms deemed to be cardiovascular in origin down to 11% of gastrointestinal symptoms (see Table 1.3).

A further possibility which was only partially explored [6] is that people self-medicate for too long because they are disillusioned by the care which they think they might receive under the auspices of the National Health Service — possibly because of an unfortunate encounter on some previous occasion. Alternatively, they may be ignorant of the severe potential of some symptoms. For whatever reasons, the attenders in our study indicated that they would be more inclined than the non-attenders to consult a doctor within a month in response to the onset and continued presence of some hypothetical symptoms (see Table 1.4).

In conclusion it can be stated that self-medication is a traditional, sensible and indeed essential component of health care and there is evidence to suggest that people are using home remedies in an effective

Table 1.4 Hypothetical general practitioner consultation (would not go to general practitioner for 1 month or more)

Hypothetical symptom	Attenders	Non-attenders
Painful swelling on calf	19%	30%
Constipation	49%	53%
Haematuria	8%	8%
Pain in chest (after walking)	32%	43%
Continuous thirst	27%	30%
Cough, fever and pain	3%	10%
Number interviewed 100%	377	300

way. There is also evidence that self-medication and requests for medical advice are, on the whole, appropriately balanced. Nevertheless there is a possibility that a few people may be self-medicating some symptoms in a potentially harmful way and that they may be continuing to treat symptoms themselves beyond the point when a medical consultation would seem to be advisable. The extent to which further research can clarify these and other issues related to self-medication is the prime reason for this conference. It is to be hoped that the exchange of information about work being undertaken and the crossfertilization of ideas in discussion will help to indicate pointers as to what needs to be done and how best to set about it.

References

1. Guthrie, D. (1945). *A History of Medicine.* (Edinburgh: Nelson)
2. Cartwright, A. (1968). *Patients and their Doctors.* (London: Routledge and Kegan Paul)
3. Anderson, J.A.D. (1975). *Gen. Pract. Int.,* **2**, 57

4. Wadsworth, M.E.J., Butterfield, W.J.H. and Blaney, R. (1971). *Health and Sickness; The Choice of Treatment.* (London: Tavistock Publications).
5. Dunnell, K. and Cartwright, A. (1972). *Medicine Takers, Prescribers and Hoarders.* (London: Routledge and Kegan Paul)
6. Anderson, J.A.D., Buck, C., Danahar, K. and Fry, J. (1977). *J. R. Coll. Gen. Practit.,* 27, 155

2

Facts and issues in self-care

D. C. MORRELL

I must initially clarify my own position and make it plain that I am not a great expert on self-care, although I have dabbled in this subject. In providing the facts for this chapter, I am dependent on the work of others and, in particular, that of Karen Dunnell and Ann Cartwright, to my knowledge the only workers to carry out a random sample survey of England and Scotland to collect information about self-care.

There are a number of ways of collecting information about self-care. I will describe below three methods with one example of each demonstrating the method and describing some of the results.

My own results stem from a study in which individuals were persuaded to keep a diary of their health on a day-to-day basis recording any illness they experienced and the action they took in response to this illness. This method is attractive in that there are no problems associated with recalling symptoms of illness, and the action taken, whether a medicine or otherwise, can be directly related to the symptoms. It is, however, expensive in that the individuals concerned need constant reminders, and the fact that their attention is focused over a period of time on their health means that a record may be biased in terms of over-recording. It is also only possible on a strictly limited geographical basis and patients must be reasonably intelligent and literate to cooperate. Nevertheless, it does provide some useful information.

The second method of obtaining information (I shall use the work of

Dunnell and Cartwright [1] to illustrate it) depends on the ability of individuals to recall the symptoms they have experienced and the action they have taken over a period of time, usually 2 to 4 weeks. Individuals may be prompted by a checklist of symptoms or they may be asked open-ended questions. It is a method which is suitable for population surveys, but main disadvantages are the dependence on memory for the recall of symptoms over a fixed time-space, and the fact that the association between symptoms experienced and the action taken is less immediate.

The third method of obtaining information is based on recording enquiries and the purchase of medicines in the pharmacy.

Table 2.1 Symptoms from the diaries of 198 patients

Symptom days (first recorded symptom)	Number
Headache	349
Changes in energy, tiredness	198
Backache	142
Cold	126
Disturbance of emotional response	98
Disturbance of gastric function	95
Sore throat	90
Abdominal pain	87
Cough	74
Pain in mouth (toothache)	55
Bleeding and abnormal discharge from nose	50
Disturbance of menstruation	48
Others	566
Total symptom days	1978

Table 2.2 Symptoms presented at 432 consultations in 1 year initiated by 198 patients keeping health diaries

Symptoms presented	Number
Sore throat	33
Cough	29
Abdominal pain	28
Skin rash	22
Disturbance of menstruation	21
Backache	21
Headache	20
Disturbance of bladder function	19
Bleeding or abnormal discharge from genital tract	15
Disturbance of bowel function	14
Chest pain	14
Disturbance of emotional response	11
Others	185
Total	432

HEALTH DIARY METHOD

This is a method of collecting information used in my practice [2], which provides care for nearly 9,000 individuals who live in the northern part of the London Borough of Lambeth. A random one-in-three sample of women aged 20—44 years were asked to record for 1 month, in a specially designed diary, symptoms they experienced and the action they took in response to these symptoms. Over a period of 1 year their requests for medical care from 'the general practitioners were recorded.

In this study, a symptom of illness was recorded on 1 day in 3, on 57% of these days on which an illness was recorded medicine was taken. By extrapolation from the monthly diaries to the annual records of requests for medical advice, it was estimated that only one symptom in 37 was reported to the general practitioner.

Table 2.1 illustrates the symptoms most commonly recorded in the diaries. As can be seen most common is headache, followed by changes in energy, backache, a cold and disturbance of emotional response (usually anxiety or depression).

Table 2.2 shows the symptoms most commonly presented to the doctor. These were, in order of frequency, sore throat, cough, abdominal pain, skin rash, etc., which suggests that patients were very discriminating in deciding which symptoms to take to the doctor. This is probably partly due to the different levels of symptom perception, different levels of anxiety provoked by different symptoms, and different expectations by the patient that the symptom perceived is appropriate to present to a doctor and is likely to be relieved by the doctors intervention.

In Table 2.4 is shown the patients' responses to some common symptoms recorded in terms of whether these restricted their activities or led to medicine-taking. Overall, 18% of symptoms led to a restriction of activities and 57% to medication, which was usually, but not exclusively, the consumption of non-prescribed medicines. The propensity to self-medicate varied with different symptoms from 78% of patients with a cough to 38% with backache or tiredness. In this study, we found that

Table 2.3 Probability of consulting in response to symptoms perceived

Symptoms episodes recorded in health diaries	Probability of consulting general practitioner
Headache	0.005
Backache	0.009
Emotional disturbance	0.012
Abdominal pain	0.026
Sore throat	0.030
Cough	0.032
All symptoms	0.027

Table 2.4 Action taken in response to ten common symptoms

Symptom days (1st recorded symptom)	Total days recorded	As a percentage of symptom days	
		Normal activities restricted	Some form of medication
Headache	349	15%	70%
Undue tiredness	198	26%	38%
Backache	142	27%	38%
'Cold' runny nose	126	24%	61%
Nerves, depression, irritability	98	21%	61%
Vomiting and indigestion	95	7%	40%
Sore throat	90	19%	59%
Abdominal pain	87	21%	53%
Cough	74	27%	78%
Toothache	55	7%	82%
Total symptom days	1978	18%	57%

self-medication was not a substitute for consultation, and that those patients who most frequently responded to symptoms by taking medicine also consulted the doctor most frequently.

In using the information in these tables I must stress that it is highly selective in that it refers only to women in the 20—44 year age group in one practice in London. Of those entered in the study, only 63% completed all the measuring instruments used in the study, which included health diaries, anxiety and depression inventories, a health and social questionnaire and a complete year of consultation data in the practice. The information I have provided about self-medication was really a byproduct of a more ambitious (some might say too ambitious) study of the factors which influence demands for general practitioner care. The main value of this information to the subsequent discussions is in the immediate way it relates symptoms perceived and recorded to the medicine taken.

SYMPTOM RECALL METHOD

In contrast to the work with health diaries, the work of Dunnell and Cartwright [1] is much more generally suited to the population at large. They studied a random sample of subjects from twelve English and two Scottish parliamentary constituencies and they depended on the subjects' recall over 24 hours and a 2 week period for the information they collected on symptom prevalence and medication. I propose to use their data as a source of information on medicine-taking.

They found that 55% of adults had taken some medicine in the 24 hours preceding the interview, and 80% during the preceding 2 weeks Women took more medicines than men, age was not closely related to medicine-taking until the age of 75, more individuals over 75 took medicines, but this was mainly due to their increased intake of prescribed medicines. In Table 2.5, I have adapted the figures from Dunnell and Cartwright to illustrate the relationship between medicine-taking and age.

In children, these workers found that under the age of two 74% of children had received a non-prescribed medicine in the 2 weeks prior to interview and this fell to 55% between the ages of two to four years.

Table 2.5 Medicine-taking in weeks prior to interview (adapted from Dunnell and Cartwright[2])

Per cent who had taken	Age groups							All adults
	21—24	25—34	35—44	45—54	55—64	65—74	Over 75	
Any medicine	75	80	80	78	80	82	92	80
Prescribed medicine	33	40	36	32	43	49	71	41
Non-prescribed medicine	67	69	71	67	64	65	71	67
Average number of medicines taken	2.1	2.0	2.1	2.1	2.2	2.7	3.2	2.2

There is, of course, a vast amount of information in the book Dunnell and Cartwright, which is impossible to completely extract, but one question they asked and to which I think we should address ourselves is 'What sort of people take medicines — prescribed or unprescribed?' They found no significant relationship between medicine-taking and social class. They did, however, find that patients with high neuroticism scores were more likely to take medicines, but these individuals were also much more likely to report symptoms. Similarly, in our work we found that patients who scored high on anxiety scales or depression inventories were more likely to record symptoms in the health diary, consult the doctor and take medicines. They found that medical knowledge or belief in the doctor's ability to cure was not related to medicine-taking. On the other hand, they found that those who were more likely to turn to the doctor for particular conditions and personal problems were more likely to take medicines.

STUDIES OF PHARMACIES

The third method of obtaining information about self-medication is derived from work in the pharmacy. Miss L. S. Boylan [3], a pharmacist working in East Anglia, recorded the enquiries for medicines for 4 days in each of ten retail pharmacies. The average number of enquiries was ten per day and altogether she was able to observe 365 enquiries about symptoms. The symptoms most commonly enquired about concerned coughs, skin conditions, gastrointestinal conditions, and requests for analgesics; 62% of all enquiries were dealt with entirely by the pharmacist and the remainder usually referred to a doctor. Most enquiries resulted in a purchase of some form of remedy but in nearly 20% of those presenting with skin disorders or gastrointestinal symptoms, the patient was given advice only and was not recommended to make a purchase.

In Table 2.6 I have compared the medicines most commonly requested or used in the three studies which I have described above. Under the work of Dunnell and Cartwright, I have divided the patients into adults and children. My own findings [2], refer, as stated above, only to women aged 20 — 44 years, which possibly accounts for the high level of psychotropic drugs taken, and this refers to the actual medicines which were recorded in the health diaries. The work of Boylan [3] covers all age and sex groups who visited the pharmacies which she was studying. The high level of demand for skin preparations which is apparent particularly

Table 2.6   Most commonly taken medicines (a comparison of three studies)

Dunnell and Cartwright		Morrell and Wale	Boylan
Adults (symptom recall)	Children (symptom recall)	Women 20—44 (diaries)	(Pharmacy observation)
Analgesics	Skin preparations	Analgesics	Throat and cough medicines
Gastrointestinal medicines	Analgesics	Psychotropics	Skin preparations
Throat and cough medicines	Throat and cough medicines	Vitamins	Gastrointestinal medicines
Skin preparations	Vitamins	Throat and cough medicines	Analgesics
	Cold 'cures'	Gastrointestinal medicines	Cold 'cures'

in Dunnell's study of children and in Boylan's study is perhaps something which is a little unexpected and which we sometimes lose sight of.

In Table 2.7 I have returned to my own study where, as I indicated, it was possible to relate the symptoms recorded in the diaries to the medicines taken on the same day and also recorded in the health diaries. It does not necessarily imply that there was always therapeutic intent, but it does, however, provide an opportunity to make some subjective assessment of the appropriateness or otherwise of the medicines consumed. In our study, we took this a stage further by inspecting individual health diaries. Again, this was a highly subjective exercise but with the exception of the use of aspirin — containing analgesics in the treatment of gastrointestinal infections, the medicine taking seemed by and large fairly rational.

THE CURRENT SITUATION IN SELF-CARE

Regarding the factors and the issues of importance in self-care, I shall try to sum up the situation as I see it. The population at large experiences many symptoms of ill-health. In my own study, one symptom of ill-health was recorded on 1 day in 3, but very few of these symptoms are reported to the general practitioner, maybe as few as one in 30. The exact figure is unimportant; what is important is that the vast majority of

Table 2.7 Type of medicine taken in response to common symptoms (from Banks *et al* [4])

Symptom recorded	Number of days	Percentage of symptom days on which medicine recorded *						
		No medicine	Vitamin	Psychotropic medicine	Gastrointestinal medicine	Respiratory medicine	Analgesic medicine	Other medicine
Headache	349	30	7	11	1	2	56	6
Undue tiredness	198	62	16	8	2	0	10	9
Backache	142	62	10	1	1	0	20	6
'Cold' runny nose	126	39	2	0	4	28	31	13
Nerves, depression, irritability	98	39	4	50	0	6	10	1
Vomiting or indigestion	95	60	2	6	23	3	12	4
Sore throat	90	41	4	6	0	16	30	20
Abdominal pain	87	47	6	2	23	21	21	1
Cough	74	22	1	0	1	54	9	28

* More than one type of medicine could be taken on any one day, therefore these totals exceed 100 per cent

symptoms are dealt with without recourse to the medical profession. Were it otherwise, the primary care services would almost certainly collapse under the demand. In other words, the basic concept of the health service as envisaged in 1948 to provide for all the medical needs of the population free of charge does not really operate. Personal responsibility in managing the many minor symptoms of illness is clearly an integral part of our health service.

Medicine-taking is clearly related to the perception of symptoms of illness. Those who record or recall a large number of symptoms are most likely to take medicine and most likely to consult the doctor. The recording and recall of symptoms is in turn related to measures of anxiety, neuroticism and depression, and a type of personality can be recognized who is more likely to perceive and report symptoms and to respond to them by taking medicine and by consulting a doctor. Medicine-taking is more common in women but is not related to social class, although there is evidence of a higher morbidity in the lower social classes, which produces more symptoms and thus a tendency to take more medicines than individuals in the higher social classes.

A significant number of individuals when faced with symptoms of illness consult the pharmacist in order to obtain medicines to treat their own symptoms. In roughly two-thirds of these, the pharmacist is able to advise and in the remainder refers the individual to a doctor. As far as I can judge from my studies and others, most self-medication is reasonably appropriate and this is presumably a result of education, either within the family, from the medical and pharmaceutical professions or from advertisements from the pharmaceutical industry.

So far, I have tried to limit myself to providing factual information based on studies of medicine-taking which have been carried out in this country. In presenting some of the issues I cannot avoid making some statements which may be regarded rather as philosophical, pragmatic or political. We must, I think, recognize that there is a built-in disincentive for individuals to treat themselves, and this is the cost of medicines. It is in fact much cheaper to consult a doctor and obtain a prescription than to visit a pharmacist and purchase a medication over the counter. When I first entered general practice in Lambeth over 10 years ago I used to send my patients to the local pharmacist when they were suffering from an upper respiratory infection with instructions to purchase a shilling's-worth of menthol crystals. About 2 years ago, the pharmacist drew my attention rather wryly to the fact that the shilling would not even purchase the paper and packaging in which the crystals were sold — but he continued to provide the patients with their shilling's worth of crystals in order to protect his goodwill and mine.

It never ceases to amaze me and I am thankful for it that so many people act responsibly in the use of general practitioner services, but I cannot see how this can continue in the face of increasing economic stringency and the desire of patients to take medicines for their symptoms. A number of possible solutions come to mind, which will be discussed in the following chapters. It would, for instance, be possible to limit the drugs which can be prescribed by the general practitioner to those which are curative, such as antibiotics, those which replace natural substances, such as hormones, and those which have dangerous side-effects, such as hypotensive drugs. Doubtless, this would cause innumerable anomalous situations, but it would have the effect of driving patients to purchase symptomatic remedies from the pharmacist. As a sequel to this, it would be possible to insist that all individuals should register with a pharmacist who should be paid a capitation fee for registration and from whom symptomatic remedies can be obtained free of charge or on payment of a nominal sum.

One of the strange features in the development of the primary care services in this country is that we have developed primary care nurses and health visitors to take more and more responsibility while the general practice pharmacist with a 3 year degree course behind him and compulsory trainee year is being relegated to the role of the shopkeeper. Something is seriously wrong here. We have in this country a great resource of highly qualified pharmacists who spend their days selling cosmetics. Is our National Health Service so well off that we can afford to throw away such resources?

We could indulge in educational programmes for school-leavers or even adult education classes in simple, symptomatic care, but there is no evidence that education helps in this field and it has no hope in the face of the present economic arguments. All the market forces are at the moment in favour of the individual obtaining a prescription for symptomatic remedies from his or her general practitioner and only doctors' appointments systems, full waiting rooms, a very acute consciousness on the part of the patients of the needs of society, or a rugged independence, act as deterrents. I do not see that these can hold up for very long with the increasing cost of medicines, and if they do not, I fear for the primary care services in this country.

References

1. Dunnell, K. and Cartwright, A. (1972). *Medicine Takers, Prescribers and Hoarders.* (London: Routledge and Kegan Paul).
2. Morrell, D. C. and Wale, C. J. (1976). Symptoms perceived and recorded by patients. *J. R. Coll. Gen. Practit.,* **26**, 398
3. Boylan, L. J. (1978). Personal communication, unpublished work for MSc degree, Bradford.
4. Banks, M. H., Beresford, S.A.A., Morrell, D. C., Waller, J. J. and Watkins, C. J.(1975). *Int. J. Epidemiol.,* **4**, 89

3

Use and misuse of home medicines

J. CROOKS and L. J. CHRISTOPHER

INTRODUCTION

A number of studies have shown that two-thirds of individuals thought that their health was poor or only fair [1, 2]. On the other hand, 'feeling unwell' is a common experience and nine out of ten adults selected at random from a large population had one or more complaints in the 2 weeks prior to being interviewed. While no medicines were taken for about half (47%) of those reporting symptoms, as expected the greater the number of symptoms the greater the use of medication [1]. With one complaint it was found that 53% of adults took self-prescribed and 43% took prescribed medicines and with four or more complaints the figures rose to 88% for self-prescribed and a similar figure for prescribed [3]. Furthermore, adults with one symptom took an average of 1.1 medicines while adults with six or more symptoms took on average four medicines [1]. Wadsworth *et al.* [2] described a higher use of self-prescribed medicines and found overall a two-fold frequency of self-prescribed to prescribed medicines. Symptoms most likely to lead to self-treatment were temperature (94%), headaches (83%), indigestion (81%) and sore throats (78%) [1]. It was reported that as many as 29% adults and 39% of children took some form of medicine even though they were not ill in any way [3].

Recent evidence therefore supports the view that symptoms of illness are often dealt with by self-treatment and a smaller number by prescribed medicines. Furthermore according to Horder and Horder [4] only a small minority of patients with symptomatic illnesses are admitted to hospital.

At first sight, examination of national annual expenditure on drugs does not appear to show a higher use of home medicines than prescribed medicines since the former is only a third of the expenditure of the latter, which incidentally was more than £500 million for 1977. However, while prescribed medicines are on average more expensive than home medicines, in terms of quantity, the latter are more frequently used but possibly more often taken in an erratic fashion [2]. In recent years the increasing cost of home medicines in contrast to the stable fee for prescribed medicines may have influenced their relative use and this merits study.

To meet the demand for home remedies an ever-widening range of medicines is available. The most recent *Martindale* (27th edition) gives details of 1450 preparations, over 80% of which are multiple-ingredient, and this list is not comprehensive. The average number of active ingredients in a sample of proprietaries from this list was 4.6 [5]. In addition, it is often not known by either the public or the medical profession that many preparations for similar indications contain similar or identical ingredients. For example, one purchaser of home medicines in a Dundee survey [6] was found to be taking four types of analgesic tablets, three of which contained paracetamol, and a total of seventeen tablets a day were taken. In such circumstances it would have been impractical for the average general practitioner to determine exactly what medicines his patient was taking, even if a history of self-medication was elicited from the patient's interview. This illustrates the fact that the avoidance of possible interactions with prescribed medicines presents a drug information problem to patient and doctor. Thus it would be reasonable to suggest that the use of complex multiple-ingredient preparations for simple symptomatic treatment should be discouraged especially when preparations with one active principle are available. While some traditional remedies probably have some valuable properties and may be useful, many depend wholly or in part on the placebo effect for their efficacy. The usefulness of the placebo effect should not, however, be underestimated and it is of interest that there is some evidence in support of a pharmacological basis for the analgesic effect produced by placebos in painful conditions [7].

About two-thirds of all medicines taken by adults in the study by Dunnell and Cartwright [1] were said to have helped. In the view of the individuals studied self-prescribed medicines were at least as efficacious as prescribed and overall this efficacy rating is better than the one-third success that could be expected as a placebo effect [8]. However, evaluation of efficacy presents great difficulties because of the subjective nature of most symptoms treated. Nevertheless efforts should be made to develop acceptable scientific methods to investigate this problem.

THE USE OF HOME MEDICINES

Much of the information regarding the use of home medicines in the United Kingdom has been derived by population surveys using electoral registers or general practitioners' lists. Such studies are expensive in time and manpower. More recently information on this subject has been derived from a study carried out by interviewing purchasers of home medicines at the time of purchase in the pharmacy [6]. While information on the incidence of use in the community was not possible, it provided a simple way of identifying home medicines actually purchased and ascertaining the attitudes of the purchasers towards their use.

In this study conducted in five Dundee pharmacies it was found that of 683 individual users there were 204 males and 479 females — a female : male ratio of 2.4:1. Children showed no sex difference but with increasing age there was an increasing female preponderance. Of the 1034 items purchased analgesics were the most popular group, comprising 27% of the total, followed by antacids (12%), laxatives (9%), antitussives (8%) and expectorants (7%).

In this survey there were eight analgesics among the top twelve preparations purchased of which four contained multiple ingredients. Paracetamol was the most common active ingredient in this group. Overall, the expectorant Benylin (4.4%) was the most popular proprietary preparation. Approximately 12% of all items bought contained an antihistamine as a constituent, mainly in cough remedies, nasal decongestants and travel sickness remedies.

Of those who bought home medicines for their own use, 80% felt that their illness was too trivial to mention to their GP and they could manage it adequately themselves; this is compatible with our finding that (after excluding first-time users) in 70% of cases self-medication was not discussed with the GP. On the other hand 36% had consulted their GP in the last month, 69% within the last year and 40% were already on prescribed medicines. Therefore users of home medicines attended their GPs with the same frequency as estimated for a sample population in previous large-scale studies [1—3].

The reason for choosing the medicine was on the users' own assessment in 30% of cases, advice from a chemist in 21%, and a doctor in 14%. The news media, the daily papers (2%) and television (2%), were only occasionally admitted by interviewees to have influenced their choice. The psychological factors that combine to produce a decision to buy a home medicine are complex, but vigorous advertising must lead to a profitable result in view of its continuing use. There is the possibility that the extent of the media's influence is erroneously low because interviewees may not readily admit to being as easily influenced by advertising as is actually the case.

Of those buying a home medicine for self-use 21% were already taking it daily for 6 months or more, and while the sex distribution was unremarkable, half (51%) were 65 years old or more, compared to 29% in this age group overall. The elderly were therefore significantly more prone to habitual use of home medicines. As expected the drugs popularly bought for continuous use were mainly antacids, analgesics and laxatives.

Of the users interviewed (excluding first-time users) only 6.6% had experienced a side-effect to the preparations bought or to a home medicine of the same group, and another 7.3% knew of side-effects or restrictions to be observed in their use. This lack of knowledge concerning side-effects may be related to the fact that many users are not aware of individual constituents of multiple-ingredient preparations, or the name of the active ingredient in single-ingredient drugs previously purchased under a different proprietary name.

THE MISUSE OF HOME MEDICINES

Misuse of home medicines may occur in a number of different situations:
(1) Drugs are taken for wrong indications or to achieve an inappropriate objective, for example, primarily to avoid the doctor;
(2) The same active ingredient may be taken in different preparations unknowingly for a given symptom;
(3) Drugs taken may interact with other home or prescribed medicines;
(4) There may be a wrong dosage; or accidental overdose, such as in children; intentional overdose; or habituation.
(5) There may be unsuitable storage conditions: light, temperature, duration, etc.

In the context of misuse of home medicines special consideration should be given to the more commonly used preparations, such as analgesics and antihistamines. The fact that many analgesics are sold as multiple-ingredient preparations may be confusing to the purchaser. In the Dundee study, of 120 who purchased analgesics for their personal use, there was a 4:1 female preponderance but age distribution was not remarkable. 12% bought 96 or more tablets; 20% had knowledge of side-effects, and 40% were taking another medication, of whom one-fifth were using another analgesic. In 7% of users taking analgesics, the indication for use did not conform with accepted practice, that is, two had purchased the analgesic for tiredness, one for insomnia, three for indigestion, one for stomach pain and one for 'kidney trouble'. While these figures appear small they must be viewed in the context of the dominant position of analgesics in the market for home medicines.

While the extent of purchases of preparations containing antihistamines was lower (50 buying for their personal use) the level of concurrent medication (44%) and the possibility of interaction (9%) were similar to the analgesics. The increasing use of this drug group is probably the outstanding difference in current sales as compared with studies of 10 years or more ago. It follows that there is an increased risk of interaction between antihistamines and alcohol or other psychotropic drugs, and this is worthy of investigation in relation to road traffic accidents and accidents in the home.

In the Dundee survey a quarter of those on prescribed medicines at the time of purchase of their home medicines could not recall the name of their prescribed medicine(s). Of those who did there was a possibiltiy of drug interaction in a quarter, although none was considered to be of an immediately serious nature. They were, as might be expected, of two main types: those where there could be an additive effect (90%) on the one hand, and on the other, those where there could be an opposing pharmacological effect (10%). An example of the former was the concurrent use of antihistamine in a nasal decongestant together with the use of a hypnotic, and of the latter, an antidiarrhoeal prepartion containing kaolin and morphine taken with a laxative, such as 'health' salts.

The way in which home medicines are stored gives rise to concern in respect of their proper use. The size of the problem is illustrated by the finding of Dunnell and Cartwright [1] of 10.3 different medicines per household in the 686 visited; there were on average three prescribed and 7.3 non-prescribed. They also found that 44% of household medicines were kept in the kitchen and 23% in the bathroom. In addition they observed that 29% of self-prescribed medicines had been in the home for a year or more and one in five of these had not been used in the past year. Recently some health authorities have carried out dump campaigns, whereby the public are asked to hand in all the tablets and other medicines they may have at home and are not in current use to special collecting centres. Such a campaign in the Tayside region yielded just under a half a tonne of medicines. The vast majority of drugs (98%) were prescribed medicines. Many aspirin tablets received had undergone hydrolization and contained free salicylic acid — a potent gut irritant. A number of tablets contained phenacetin, withdrawn from the market 4 years ago because of its association with serious renal disease. Many antibiotics had outlasted their shelf-life and some sulphonamide tablets had been long off the market and were among the earliest of the sulphonamides used (sulphathiazols and sulphapyridine, for instance).

It was obvious from the survey that the public often hoard medicines. In the light of the figures of Dunnell and Cartwright [1] it is surprising that only 2% of medicines returned were home medicines. This is similar to the figure returned in a Manchester dump campaign and not far removed from 6.3% found in Glasgow [9, 10]. Perhaps home medicines are more confidently used by the average person who may use just the minimum of prescribed medicines. Are we over-prescribing? Is there a high degree of non-compliance to prescribed medicines? Do patients visit their GPs for the purpose of discussing their problems rather than to get pills? Whatever the reasons may be, and they certainly require further investigation, the hoarding of prescribed medicines in the home allows the individual to self-treat with the prescribed medicines retained in the household from any previous medically treated illness.

CONCLUSIONS

The conclusions arrived at, based on the literature reviewed in this paper and on the Dundee survey [6], are as follows:

(1) The occurrence of symptoms is very common in the community at large and is related to the extensive use of home medicines.
(2) The range of home medicines available is wide, perhaps unduly so particularly in the case of multiple-ingredient preparations. The analgesics continue to be the dominant group, while preparations containing antihistamines are increasing in popularity.

(3) The benefits of self-medication although difficult to measure, appear, in the majority of instances to justify their use. A component of this benefit is likely to be a placebo effect, the value of which should not be underestimated.

(4) The extent of misuse of home medicines does not appear too large although certain problem areas have been identified, for example, lack of knowledge of indications and side-effects, reliability of sources of relevant information, long-term use, unsatisfactory storage, drug interactions and lack of communication with the general practitioner.

A number of the problems identified have been considered by a working group of the Council of Europe (European Public Health Community) [11], who cite some basic rules to which the public should adhere if self-medication is to be responsible and safe:

(1) Take care with any medicine, however harmless it may appear to be.
(2) Always read carefully the direction folder provided with a medicine.
(3) Never treat any symptom for longer than a week without consulting your doctor.
(4) If a medicine which you have used according to instructions fails to have the desired effect, consult your doctor.
(5) Only treat young children with medicines which are specifically stated on the packaging to be suitable for them.
(6) Do not take any medicines during pregnancy or breastfeeding without your doctor's advice.
(7) If you are being treated by a doctor, do not, without consulting him, take any medicines other than those which he has prescribed for you, even medicines prescribed by another doctor.
(8) Keep medicines in a closed, dark cupboard in a cool place, out of the reach of children.
(9) Do not keep medicines for longer than a year.
(10) *Destroy completely* what is left of a medicine after you have finished with it. *Never throw medicines into the dustbin.*

References

1. Dunnell, K. and Cartwright, A. (1972). *Medicine Takers, Prescribers and Hoarders.* (London: Routledge and Kegan Paul)

2. Wadsworth M.E.J., Butterfield, W.J.H. and Blaney R. (1971). *Health and Sickness: The Choice of Treatment* (London: Tavistock Publications).
3. Jefferys, M., Brotherston, J. H. F. and Cartwright, A. (1960). Consumption of medicines on a Working Class Housing Estate. *Br. J. Prev. Soc. Med.,* **14**, 64
4. Horder, J. and Horder, E. (1954). Illness in general practice. *Practitioner,* **173**, 177
5. *Martindale: The Extra Pharmacopeia,* ed. W. Aimley (London: The Pharmaceutical Press)
6. Christopher, L. J., Crooks, G. and Kilgallon, B. *Dundee Survey on Self-Medication* (unpublished)
7. Levine, J. D., Gordon, N. C. and Fields, H. L. (1978). The mechanism of placebo analgesia. *Lancet,* **ii**, 654
8. Beecher, H. K. J. (1955). The powerful placebo. *J. Am. Med. Assoc.,* **159**, 1602
9. Bradley, T. J. and William, W. H. (1975). Evaluation of medicines returned in Manchester dump campaign. *Pharm. J.,* **215**, 542
10. Sixsmith, D. G., Smail, G. A. (1978). Evaluation of medicines returned in Glasgow dump campaign. *Health Bull.,* **36**(2), 88
11. Report by a Working Party, Council of Europe, European Public Health Community (1976). *Abuse of Medicines Part I. Self-Medication, Drug Intelligence and Clinical Pharm.,* **10**, 16

Supplementary discussion — points for consideration

1. The cost of home medicines has been rising, whereas the prescription fee has remained stable. What is the influence of this on the use of home medicines?
2. Is it feasible to assess the effect of home medicines including the placebo effect by the application of scientific methods, such as clinical trials?
3. What is the case for and against the use of multiple-ingredient preparations in the field of home medicines?
4. What are the implications which follow from the fact that long-term use of home medicines is not uncommon, particularly in the elderly?
5. There appears to be a lack of knowledge of side-effects and restrictions to be observed in the use of home medicines. What are the consequences and what action is necessary?
6. What measures are required to improve the safe and effective storage of home medicines?

Supplementary discussion

Chairman: R. Goulding
Prime discussant: T. G. Stewart
Rapporteur: J. B. Spooner

There was no dispute by the group of the basic conclusions of Crooks and Christopher that the benefits of self-medication appear in the majority of instances to justify its use and that the extent of misuse of home medicines does not appear too large. They also gave in their conclusions a number of qualifying statements and identified areas where knowledge on the use and misuse of home medicines is limited. These were presented to the Group in the form of a series of questions.

(1) *The cost of home medicines has been rising, whereas the prescription fee has remained stable. What is the influence of this on the use of home medicines?*

The average cost of a small pack of home medicines is about 40p to 50p and the rate of increase in this cost in recent years has in general been less than the increase in the retail price index.

The prescription fee at 20p per item has remained unchanged for several years and was considered to be essentially a political gesture. When the fee was increased there was a slowing down in the rate of increase in the number of prescription medicines dispensed, but this effect soon disappeared and the increasing rate was resumed.

The general conclusion of the Group was that the modest cost of home medicines does not act as a significant deterrent to their purchase and an encouragement to obtain a supply of equivalent prescription medicines through the NHS. It was considered that the inconvenience of visiting the general practitioner and having the medicine dispensed at a pharmacy normally outweighed the modest cost saving to the individual. Furthermore, consumers are not always particulary cost-conscious when purchasing medicines, provided they obtain value for money in terms of an adequate therapeutic response.

The Group identified two possible areas where this generalization may not apply. The first is the individual with a chronic recurring simple symptom, such as dysmenorrhoea, where benefit may be derived by obtaining a prescription with an adequate supply of medicine to cover 6 months requirements.

The second is the pensioner who is exempt from the prescription charge and who has more time to visit his general practitioner or indeed may add a request for a prescription during the course of a consulation for some other reason.

The extent to which either of these possibilities occurs has not been investigated, and the Group considered that it would be worthwhile doing so, taking into account also the total cost to the NHS of such 'trivial' consultations.

The Group concluded that at present the cost of home medicines compared with the cost to the individual of prescription medicines has a minimal influence on the use of home medicines, but that an investigation into the relationship, if any, between increasing home medicine costs and an unchanged prescription fee could be carried out to determine whether there comes a point where the difference significantly alters the way medicines are obtained. In such an investigation special subgroups such as old age pensioners should be studied.

(2) *Is it feasible to assess the effect of home medicines including the placebo effect by the application of scientific methods, such as clinical trials?*

The Group generally agreed that it would be extremely difficult to carry out an evaluation of home medicines under the conditions of their normal use because of the many factors that influence an individual's decision to take a home medicine and which influence the response. In addition the placebo response is an important aspect of the value of home medicines, particularly since these medicines are essentially for the relief of subjective symptoms rather than the cure of disease, and this would need to be taken into account in the assessment of benefit.

It was thought important, however, to have some clinical evidence by scientific methods of the therapeutic activity of the ingredients of home medicines not only in terms of efficacy, but also to investigate

41

side-effects. The latter are particularly important since safety is the absolute prerequisite of home medicines.

The scientific evaluation of the mechanism of the placebo response was considered a topic more suitable to investigation under controlled clinical situations than directly in regard to home medicines.

The Group concluded that it is not feasible to assess the effect of home medicines by the application of scientific methods, but that an indication of the activity of these medicines could be achieved by scientific study of their active ingredients.

(3) *What is the case for and against the use of multiple-ingredient preparations in the field of home medicines?*

There was a general distrust of multiple-ingredient home medicines — the argument being that they are no more effective than single-ingredient preparations and yet carry a greater potential for unwanted effects.

In their support, it was suggested that some minor illnesses of everyday life present a cluster of symptoms for which a single ingredient would not be adequate and therefore the individual would have to take more than one preparation to obtain relief. Such multiple-product consumption carries the risks of choice of the wrong medicines, drug interactions and inappropriate dosage. Such problems do not arise with the multiple-ingredient preparations specifically developed for that situation.

It was also suggested that two ingredients with the same therapeutic effect, though often with different pharmacological actions, may be able to provide better effect than a single ingredient, or greater safety because smaller doses can be given to produce the same effect.

The Group concluded that the use of multiple-ingredient home medicines should be discouraged when single-ingredient preparations are available and capable of producing the desired therapeutic response, but that there may be a place for multiple-ingredient preparations where the ingredients are limited to two or three and a rational basis for the combination exists, such as a demonstrated additive effect or action against a cluster of symptoms.

(4) *What are the implications that follow from the fact that long-term use of home medicines is not uncommon, particularly in the elderly?*

Although data were presented by Crooks and Christopher that 21% of those buying a home medicine for self-use were already taking it daily for 6 months or more and that 51% of these people were 65 years old or more, the Group considered that there was insufficient information available in respect of the circumstances of this use to be able to draw conclusions. For example, was the continuing use of these preparations based on an earlier medical recommendation?

However, the Group considered that this was potentially a cause for concern, as it was felt that no patient should continue on the same medicaiton, prescribed or purchased, without a clinical review at least every 6 months.

The Group concluded that the long-term use of home medicines, particularly in the elderly, is a subject that requires specific investigation in order to determine its extent and the circumstances under which it is carried out. Limitations on the duration of use of home medicines should be considered if a real problem is identified by this investigation.

(5) *There appears to be a lack of knowledge of side-effects and restrictions to be observed in the use of home medicines. What are the consequences and what action is necessary?*

Two points of view were expressed on the need to provide consumers with information on specific side-effects of home medicines. One was that the provision of such information is unhelpful, since the incidence of significant side-effects to home medicines is very small and all that would be achieved would be an encouragement to anticipate the specified side-effect; it might also have a negative effect on the placebo response.

The second view was that the consumer should be in possession of side-effect information in order to make an informed decision as to whether or not to take that medicine.

There appears to be no factual evidence to support either point of view in terms of patient benefit and the Group therefore agreed that there is a need for an investigation into the incidence, nature and severity of side-effects to home medicines in order to decide whether a need exists in terms of providing consumers with information on side-effects.

It was considered that restrictions to be observed in the use of home medicines should be those appropriate to the majority of users. The Medicines Act (1968) requires a number of warning statements, such as keeping the product out of the reach of children, to be included on labelling. Such non-medical statements appear to cover all the current problem areas and the Group considered that medical restrictions, such as the use of aspirin by haemophiliacs, were not appropriate restrictions to be referred to on home medicine labelling, but should be an important advisory role for the general practitioner. A possible exception concerned a common situation where a particular medicine would be inappropriate such as the use of aspirin for the relief of stomach pain.

The Group concluded that there is no adequate information on the effect of the apparent lack of knowledge on side-effects by consumers though no problem resulting from it was clearly identified. It was agreed that an investigation into the incidence, nature and severity of side-effects to home medicines would be desirable so that a decision could be made as to what, if anything should be communicated to consumers on this topic.

It was further concluded that the restrictions to be observed in the use of home medicines are at present largely adequately conveyed to the consumer.

(6) *What measures are required to improve the safe and effective storage of home medicines?*

Since accidental ingestion and poisoning with home medicines is very rare, it was felt that home medicines are being adequately stored to provide safety from this form of misuse. Such storage includes the use of strip and blister and other child-resistant packaging.

All home medicines are required to declare their shelf-life if this is less than three years. Since home medicines are largely purchased for immediate or recurring needs, the possibility of the product being kept long enough for significant deterioration to take place and for the product to be subsequently consumed is extremely small.

Furthermore, home medicines are sold in their original manufacturers packs which are tested for the stability of their contents under various conditions including high humidity, so that effective storage can readily be achieved in all households. Lack of safety from improper storage of home medicines is therefore unlikely.

The Group concluded that there are no additional measures required to improve the safe and effective storage of home medicines. Hoarding of home medicines does not seem to be a significant problem but the public should be encouraged not to keep large stocks for prolonged periods.

4

Home medicines — communication, advertising and education

G. CUST and
J. P. WELLS

INTRODUCTION

In 1968 a Royal Commission studying the future of the National Health Service [1] included the recommendation:

> When adequate arrangements for health education and prophylaxis have been established, the typical patient of the future — who will be better educated and better informed about health dangers — can be expected to take more responsibility for the management of trivial and self-limiting complaints, provided he is given the necessary encouragement and guidance by the medical profession: help in this respect may well be given in the course of normal schooling and in adult education.

The responsible use of home medicines is dependent upon a number of decisions which must be taken by the individual experiencing any departure from normal health. Of these varied decisions the most important involve:

(1) the recognition of symptoms suitable for self-care;
(2) when appropriate, the choice and proper use of a suitable medication.

Other chapters deal with the current practices of self-medication. This chapter considers the influence upon these decisions of information provided to the lay user on the labels of home medicines, through their advertising in the general media and through health information campaigns. In each case the authors attempt to evaluate the ability and limitations of these various methods of communicating information to assist the choice and use of home medicines and improve the quality of decision.

THE USE OF HOME MEDICINES — AIMS AND OBJECTIVES

The general aim of any educational programme in self-treatment should be to help a greater proportion of the population to deal with minor illness without bothering their general practitioners and without coming to harm. As such, the use of home medicines is only part of the much wider uses of self-care including good eating habits, proper exercise, proper hygiene, the avoidance of obesity and the abuse of alcohol and tobacco.

If the lay public are to make informed choices about self-treatment, the degree of knowledge required may be grouped under four headings: medical diagnosis, conditions for self-treatment, use of home medicines, and general health information.

Medical diagnosis

There are a number of signs and symptoms which should *always* result in a visit to the doctor for diagnosis and possible treatment, such as post-menopausal bleeding, or a lump in the breast. Consideration needs to be given to a 'key list' of symptoms requiring referral to general practitioners and the means of improving public awareness.

Conditions suitable for self-treatment

There is a need for reminding the public of conditions such as coughs, sore throats, headaches, muscular aches and pains, etc., which are suitable for self-treatment.

Use of home medicines

There is a need for detailed guidance on the choice and use of home medicines including their dosage, precautions in use, and limitations.

General health information

The lay public require general information and education on health matters. This information would include the appreciation that not all illness requires medication (either prescribed or non-prescribed), how to store medicines safely in the home, and the need to use medicines in accordance with instructions, etc.

There are a number of opportunities to provide information on the choice and use of home medicines. Firstly, there is provision of information associated with the use and purchase of a home medicine itself. In addition there are opportunities for people to acquire fresh knowledge through the normal learning process about health and illness, together with specific health education campaigns. It must be appreciated, though, that learning involves not only the desire and ability to impart information but — to be successful — also requires the willingness and ability of the recipient to understand the information provided and take the necessary action. Consequently it is essential to ensure that information is only provided at a time relevant to the person concerned and in a manner that is suitable and readily understandable by the lay person.

THE CHOICE AND USE OF A HOME MEDICINE

The use of a home medicine follows three stages — product awareness, product purchase and product use. At each of these stages there is a different information need.

Product awareness

The public become aware of the existence of a product through a variety of sources. Most commonly the choice of home medicines is based upon family experience. In most families there are well-regarded home medicines that are used for particular temporary minor ailments; having found a medicine which serves a particular need, a family is reluctant to consider alternative treatments. Indeed, of all purchases of home medicines, more than 90% are of products that have been used previously [2].

However, information about the treatment of minor illness also comes from doctors, pharmacists, nurses, health-related features and articles in the media, and advertising. The latter is particularly important in that it serves as a constant reminder both of the symptoms suitable for treatment by self-medication and of the products available. But an advertisement can do no more than draw attention to a product and perhaps generate sufficient interest for a person to consider that product when next they suffer from the symptoms it is designed to relieve. By their very nature, advertisements can effectively convey only a limited number of simple ideas, such as the name of the product and its major indications. The message is seen or heard only briefly, and complex and detailed information cannot be conveyed.

The consumer tends to remember just one thing from an advertisement — one strong claim, or one strong concept . . .
The advertisement may have said five, ten, or fifteen things, but the consumer will tend to pick out just one, or else, in a fumbling confused way, he tries to fuse them together into a concept of his own . . .
A President of the United States, while running for office, covered fourteen different points in one of his speeches. It was a clear and vigorous speech. Despite its clearness, however, a study made the next day showed that less than 2% of the people knew what he had said. Had he picked one point of focus, he might have had 30%, 40% or 50% remember the substance of his message.' [3].

While the prime function of advertising is to remind lay persons of symptoms suitable for treatment and home medicines available, it is possible for some contribution to be made to health education. Advertisements can carry simple health education messages. Since 1976 PAGB member companies have, from time to time, included the messages 'Use medicines properly' or 'Keep medicines safely' in press advertising as part of a campaign with the Health Education Council. There is the opportunity to develop other short and pertinent statements such as 'Always read the label' or 'If symptoms persist consult a doctor'.

In carrying out its function of drawing attention to conditions suitable for self-medication and the products available, advertising does much to define the proper area of self-medication. In most countries the content of advertisements is governed either by legislation or industry codes of standards. These controls invariably include the requirement that advertising should be limited to conditions suitable for self-medication.

In the UK a serious attempt has been made to define the precise areas for self-medication through the introduction of the Medicines (Labelling and Advertising to the Public) Regulations. The regulations work on this principle, and prohibit all advertising of a medicine, except for

Table 4.1

System or part of the body	Adverse conditions of those symptoms	Purposes for which advertising is permitted
1. The cardiovascular system	(a) All diseases of the myocardium and heart valves, including rheumatic heart disease and coronary artery disease	None
	(b) Hypertension	None
	(c) Thrombosis	None
	(d) Oedema	None
	(e) Peripheral artery disease	Treatment of chilblains

conditions expressly exempted in the schedules to the regulations. Table 4.1 above, showing a typical entry, gives an idea of the way the system works.

The regulations have been drafted in an attempt to limit the offer of medicines sold directly to the public to the treatment of those conditions which are self-limiting and not susceptible to a medical diagnosis. This approach derives directly from the industry codes which were compiled with particular relation to the offer of products in advertisements. The regulations are more broadly based and also limit the indications which may be included on the labels of medicines sold over the counter in pharmacies. If pharmacists are to expand their role in the supply of medicines for 'maintenance therapy' of diagnosed conditions, such as arthritic conditions, the regulations would not provide for the supply of appropriately labelled products.

Product purchase

While the majority of purchases of a medicine are made by people who have used the product in the past, pharmacists are frequently consulted about the appropriate treatment of unfamiliar symptoms and the medicines available. Questions are currently being raised in the pharmaceutical journals about the extent to which a pharmacist is equipped to answer these questions through his training. There seems opportunity to provide pharmacists with a new source of information on the recognition of common ailments and the medicines available.

A prime source of information on the use and composition of a medicine is the product label. United Kingdom legislation requires that the *outer carton* should provide the following information:

(1) Name of product
(2) Pharmaceutical form
(3) Composition (must be the wording at the head of the monograph; must be in English where possible; must be followed by the monograph initials).
(4) Quantity in containers
(5) Directions for use
(6) Contraindications (where these are required by the licence)
(7) Special handling/storage (where these are required by the licence)
(8) Expiry date (if less than 3 years)
(9) Name and address of licence holder
(10) Licence number
(11) Batch reference
(12) 'Keep out of the reach of children'

It will be seen that through reference to this outer package label the potential user can ensure that the medicine is not 'contraindicated' for the particular person contemplating purchase.

Product use

The detailed guidance on the use of a product includes all relevant dosage instructions and the cautionary statements and advice necessary to ensure the safe and correct use of the medicine. This information is best included on the inner label, remembering that home medicines are often kept in the medicine cupboard and may be used by the family at different times. It is for this reason that UK legislation demands that all the relevant information about the use of the product should be repeated on the inner label as well as being included on the outer carton.

While all will support the view that the label must provide all necessary information on the safe and proper use of the medicine, the basic requirements for 'communication' stated earlier in this paper must still apply — the information must be expressed in terms readily understood by a layman. It must also be remembered that the more detailed the information the more chance that essential guidance will be overlooked.

HEALTH EDUCATION PROGRAMMES

In devising a health education programme there are certain steps which must be taken.

(1) Targets
(2) Aims and objectives
(3) Methods

Targets

An education programme can be aimed at the whole public but as certain sections may already have adequate knowledge, concentration on specific targets may lead to a more effective programme. What area of the public needs health education? A considerable proportion of the public deal adequately with their trivial illnesses themselves, and probably need no further education on this topic.

The 'public' consist of many groups, the old, the young, men and women, different socioeconomic groups, etc. There are probably social class differences in behaviour about self-medication and it is important to know about this, as the educational messages will need to be differently designed for different social classes. The existing beliefs, attitudes and knowledge of the public about self-treatment of minor illnesses must be an essential base on which to build an educational programme, for example, the labelling of aspirin 'for symptomatic reduction of transient fever as in 'flu' may be a good message for people in the professional and managerial classes, but would fail to be understood by unskilled workers as its reading difficulty level is too high. If older schoolchildren are to be a target then material would need to be included in the health education curriculum in schools. The above examples give an idea of the complexity of education programmes.

Aims and objectives

Of the aims and objectives stated earlier, general health education programmes are probably best equipped to improve knowledge about:

(1) Symptoms suitable for self-treatment and those requiring medical attention;
(2) Generally good practice in the use of medicines and attitudes to illness, for example: store safety, read instructions, do not take medicines unnecessarily.

Methods

Person-to-person health education of the public by doctors and pharmacists would be the most important factor in any health education programme on self-medication. Doctors are trusted advisers and over the course of about 5 years see maybe 90% of the patients on their lists. Many doctors would see positive benefits in educating patients in the use of home medicines. The doctor's waiting room or clinic can be a source of posters or leaflets reinforcing professional advice.

Judicious use of a mix of mass media advertising would help to bring basic messages to a wide range of the public. There could also be a need for some supporting material in the form of a simply written self-help booklet which could be used for reference by patients, distributed through family doctors, pharmacists and health education units of AHAs. More detailed information about the specific home medicine — nature and uses, dosage, unwanted effects and storage — is best provided at the point of sale, with the home medicine or as a package leaflet.

References

1. Great Britain. (1978). Royal Commission on Medical Education 1965 to 1968: Report (Chairman The Lord Todd) (London: HMSO)
2. European Health Panel. (1977). Study in Germany and France April 1967 to March 1977, Gesellschaft für Konsum-, Markt- und Absatzforschung, Nuremburg
3. Reeves, R. (1961). Reality in Advertising. (New York: Knopf)

Supplementary discussion — points for consideration

(1) What are the educational, social and psychological characteristics of those people who,

    (a) treat their own minor illnesses
    (b) bring their trivial illnesses to their GP,
    (c) avoid any contact with their GP?

(2) What do the public know, believe, and do about minor illnesses in 1979?

(3) What should be the aims and objectives of an educational programme to promote better home medication?

(4) What harm could occur because of an increase in home medication?

(5) What signs and symptoms should always lead to medical consultation?

(6) How can we decide the minor illnesses (signs and symptoms) that are suitable for home medication?

(7) What simple short message could be contained in the advertising of medicines to supplement Health Education Campaigns — for example 'Read the label', 'if symptoms persist consult a doctor', etc.

(8) What steps should be taken to help distinguish generic and brand names for drugs?

(9) Should Area Health Authorities assume responsibility for disseminating information about prescribed drugs and their interaction with home medicines?

Supplementary discussion

Chairman: M. J. Linnett
Prime discussants: J. M. Atkinson and A. Herxheimer
Rapporteur: A. J. Hedley

INTRODUCTION

Since many of the topics raised in the questions posed by Cust and Wells overlap it was decided to place them in the context of a cycle of activities. (See Figure 4.1).

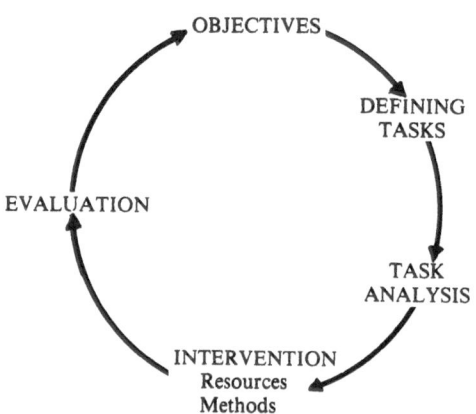

Figure 4.1

(1) setting objectives,
(2) defining tasks,
(3) task analysis,
(4) intervention (including resources, content and methods),
(5) evaluation

SETTING OBJECTIVES

The first principal discussant began by emphasizing the need to examine the issues of communication, advertising and education within the whole context of self-care and not just self-medication. Self-medication may provide a very useful model in which to study some of the important problems which must be faced in order to promote self-care (where this is wanted and needed), but self-medication must not be viewed as a discrete process in isolation from other aspects of self-care. The group agreed that there was a great deal which needed to be done on the patient's behalf in traditional encounters between health personnel (not least doctors) and patients. These include:

(1) Intelligible explanations about the nature of illness, body functions and available solutions to problems;
(2) Adequate instructions about the use of drugs.

Many references were made in one way or another to the acquisition of medical knowledge by the patients; these emphasized in particular existing deficiencies and professional barriers which tend to hinder this process. The group appeared to be supporting the acquisition of medical knowledge *inspite of the fact* that in many hospitals medical record folders still carry, in heavy black type, the *cuveat* 'Not to be handled by the patient'. As a preliminary to the setting of objectives it is worthwhile recording a definition of the self-care process. There are several available. Self-care can be viewed as a decision-making process which includes self-observation, symptom perception and labelling, judgement of severity and choice and assessment of treatment options. It is a process 'whereby a layperson functions on his or her own behalf in health promotion and prevention and in disease detection and treatment at the level of the primary health resource in the health care system' [1]. Fry [2] identified four roles for self-care which include health maintenance, disease prevention, self-diagnosis, self-medication, self-treatment and participation in professional care (use of services).

Self-care, including self-medication, is a voluntary, self-limited, relatively non-organized, universal and varying complex of behaviour patterns. It is salutary to acknowledge that it is into this somewhat complex and amorphous setting that there is a wish to intrude and to take a professional rather than a lay initiative. Implicit in the function of a multidisciplinary workshop is the need to establish a *theoretical framework* for action, within which innovations can be begun. There is thus a potential conflict in that these innovations usually stem from professional groups and therefore the general desire to deprofessionalize many aspects of the process of medication continues to be arrested.

OBJECTIVES

The primary objectives for new activity in this field can be expressed as follows:

(1) The identification of important target groups; that is, those who will benefit most from the promotion of self-care;

(2) The design and dissemination of appropriate information about the use of drugs for the treatment of common symptoms.

The objectives would appear to be entirely consistent with the recommendations adopted by the Alma Ata International Conference on Primary Health Care in 1978, particularly recommendation no. 14 on essential drugs for primary health care [3].

The secondary objectives which might be associated with these activities include:

(1) The identification and explicit classification of those common symptom complexes towards which the self-care process could be directed;

(2) The design and testing of sets of information and packaged medicines which best meet the needs of the lay public (taking into account the variability of levels of secondary educational attainment, basic levels of literacy and numeracy and linguistic/ cultural differences);

(3) The identification of the resources which can be used in promoting education programmes for the consumer — both for new information about medication and self-care and the reinforcement of existing information.

DEFINITION OF TASKS

The group agreed that further work is needed to define more clearly those bodily states which different groups of patients consider to be an illness and to identify at which stage the patient makes a decision to treat and medicate himself. Health personnel frequently overlook the fact that self-care does not, by and large, operate within the framework of professional practices and lay people do not use professional criteria to assess their own wellbeing or social competence. A most important task is the educational process and it is quite clear that unwarranted assumptions are frequently made that the lay public has assimilated knowledge about health risks and health care when frequently this is not the case [4].

One of the surveys quoted in the discussion to support this contention concerns a widespread lack of awareness about the possible effects of smoking on the outcome of a pregnancy [5]. A better understanding is needed about the ways in which lay people, at different levels of secondary educational attainment acquire knowledge about health. Some of these sources are known or self-evident, such as the family, articles in women's magazines, books written by doctors for lay use and media programmes (television and radio).

In using information derived from the family, many individuals are mimicking what they have been exposed to during their most formative years. Amongst sources available for later acquisition of information, articles in popular magazines (such as *Cosmopolitan*) are rated highly; 'doctors books' are less good in terms of their availability and intelligibility while media programmes probably rank lowest as a useful source of *balanced information*. Certainly if television is watched as little by the general population (and as apologetically) as it is by this discussion group then it is unlikely to make much impact in any sphere!

At this stage a warning was sounded about the whole issue of the medication of health as opposed to ill-health. For example, fewer people will admit to being 'fed up' or bored, but they will admit to depressive symptoms perhaps because they see a depressive state as one which is culturally acceptable and pharmacologically soluble; at least that is implicit in the actions taken by their doctors. Patients are conditioned continuously to expect medication for any complaint and this attitude may be strongly reinforced by articles in the popular press. The 'medication of health' may (if it is not already) become the prime drive for self-medication and there is a danger that as well as the assumption of responsibility self-medication may be (or may become) a major iatrogenic problem.

A programme which promotes self-medication for all psychosocial problems is something to avoid. A proper understanding of this complex problem is fundamental to any planning, by health personnel or lay public, on intervention and promotion in the field of self-medication.

TASK ANALYSIS

Information upon which to base a task analysis of the next steps in the design and promotion of educational material on self-medication is meagre but some background information which should be considered was produced. For example it was pointed out that the use of *medicines available* (OTC) is static or declining slightly; the hypochondriacs (it was asserted) are in the doctor's surgery and not in the chemists's shop. The pharmacists believe that home medicine users are a stable group and as such one whose habits and attitudes are difficult to influence. This stability, it was suggested, is recognized by the pharmaceutical industry whose advertising/promotional activities are relatively small because of the recognition that trends in the use of non-prescription medicines change very slowly. It seems however that caution is needed about the interpretation of trends in the use of OTC's and using these data to gauge the possible effects of any purposeful form of intervention such as the promotion of self-care. It is, for example, difficult to calculate rates for OTC use without a valid denominator. The latter is defined as the true population at risk of using OTC, in other words, those with symptoms. In the United States studies have shown that 'an individual's chance of being totally symptom-free on any given day is remote' [4]; some form of illness is the statistical norm, therefore [6]. But there are no good data on how such common symptoms are distributed in terms of severity. The denominator may be much larger than is suspected from actual OTC use and a change in behaviour which might be induced by combined professional and lay intervention may therefore be dramatic.

The group has asked what clues there were from general practice which might help to describe the educational processes which are needed both for the lay public and health personnel to promote the sensible use of home medicines. It was pointed out that there have been many experiments, mostly by general practitioners, aimed at trying to break patients' expectations of the doctor-initiated medication cycle. For example, on Teesside a practice group had given notice that prescriptions would not necessarily be issued for some common symptoms. The results of this action were a mixture of acceptance and antagonism on the part of patients [7]. One important problem to be faced is the possible consequence of attempts by the health professions to intervene by promoting opportunities for self-medication and thus deprofessionalizing many therapeutic processes. In this way a support may be removed from those patients who rely upon a kind of medical priesthood. Increased emphasis on self-care may not help them and may even do harm if they seek less desirable alternatives. In this context it was agreed that the term 'trivial illnesses' are things which happen to other people (rather like minor operations). When experienced personally, of course, they assume a different perspective! Above all, the promotion of self-medication for common symptoms should not become a means of protecting health personnel, for example, during unsocial hours. In the Teesside study the availability and quality of practice consultation with every member of the primary care team clearly increased.

INTERVENTION

(i) Resources

The available resources appear to be:

(1) traditional health personnel and routine health care contacts;
(2) members of other disciplines such as psychologists and educationists;
(3) existing educational processes and the media;
(4) lay people;
(5) money.

It is likely to take a good deal of the last-mentioned resource to make rapid progress in this field though, of course, considerable savings may accrue if the promotion of self-care is recognized as a legitimate target for the reallocation of resources. In terms of the content and methods which should be used for intervention, sound recommendations will only be arrived at through properly designed scientific studies. Clearly the first step should be unambitious and in the first instance we should learn to do a little well.

The harnessing of available resources means, above all, the education (and perhaps motivation) of health personnel and particularly of doctors. There is uncertainty as to how much the medical profession will do towards the promotion of this or any aspect of self-care. Some portents are not encouraging* one discussant pointed out that the term 'doctor' meant 'teacher'; doctors are not doing enough to help people to look after themselves, even with the assistance of medical care. The question 'what has the patient learned or not learned' should be asked more often on completion of any kind of routine consultation. Once the educators of health personnel are armed with adequate guidelines and perhaps teaching materials, much greater emphasis can be placed on the promotion of self-care during the training of new general practitioners, health visitors, community nurses and other caring professions. Better collaboration between different disciplines *during* their training would create more opportunities for the discussion and expansion of ideas on appropriate content and methods. The promotion of selected ideas and issues by Area Health Authorities would seem to be a rational approach, for example, through the machinery of an Area Health Education Unit and other lines of communication open to health education officers.

The education of lay people presents a special challenge which we have hardly begun to meet. Some limited success would seem likely with groups of strongly motivated adults, perhaps through adult education classes. (programmes issued by the Workers Educational Association in one locality during the last three years did not reveal any on health or health care). Educational programmes should be directed at those groups which are likely themselves to have the biggest influence on others, that is the attitude-formers. In the long term education in the earliest and most formative years of life will yield the best response. Little has been done so far, but some health education in schools has been evaluated and shown to be effective. Those children exposed to two or three modules on health and its maintenance have shown a 5 year reduction in the expected numbers who are smoking [8]. School sessions on health could lay greater emphasis on medicines, their choice and use. The importance of children as an educational resource was emphasized, particularly their ability to influence their parent's behaviour, for example, in attitudes towards and patterns of smoking. Other obvious groups include mothers with young children.

---

* Such as the comments attributed to a BMA spokesman which were reported in one newspaper, when a self-measuring device for blood-pressure was deployed for public use. His comment was that this could be hazardous as a falsely low reading might be obtained if the subject had recently sustained a silent myocardial infarction!

(ii) Methods

There was only a brief discussion on methods which revealed areas of ignorance and lack of expertise. Our objectives are agreed — so why is it not happening now? Perhaps this is because a system for the education and continuing education of different subgroups has not been worked out, that is, those with different information needs, amongst the general population tend to receive the same input. There seems to be good evidence for that need; for example, it is known that many consumers do not read or act upon those instructions which are already offered for the use of medicines. The problem may be soluble by using different instructional techniques, but the behaviour of many health personnel and their apparent difficulty in complying with recommendations when given a specific course of medication indicates that the issue may be more subtle and difficult than might at first be supposed.

EVALUATION

Checklists, decision-trees and 'consensus' information

In looking for some specific examples of decision-making processes (which is where instructional efforts must be directed) note was taken of a number of relevant experiments. For example, doctors have attempted to provide receptionists with checklists for the purpose of screening patients, but there remains a need to know more about how well this attempt at special communication between professional and lay groups works in practice.

Logical decision-trees have been developed to fit many diagnostic and therapeutic situations; for example, frontline health workers in third world countries [9], paramedical and nursing personnel in the United States and also the lay public (for example, the American publication *How to Take Care of Yourself*). The decision nodes in such logical decision-making processes must of course look beyond medication and its use. They should examine non-medication alternatives which, to illustrate the point, might include:

(1) a walk in the fresh air for headaches;
(2) humidification of centrally heated air for upper respiratory symptoms;
(3) a sheet of blockboard for a sagging bed and backache;
(4) unprocessed bran and other fibre-rich foods for constipation.

However, the task of drawing up adequate guidelines on self-management in certain conditions, for example, whether to seek medical help or not, looks difficult. Nevertheless protocols could be devised for common symptoms which are associated with self-limiting conditions, using the duration of symptoms as one of the most important criteria for the termination of self-care. The approach *must* be empirical, not diagnosis-orientated but problem and therapy-orientated.

During the preliminary discussion of the paper by Fryers when the problem of giving adequate guidance was raised, a lay member of the audience asked why sulphacetamide ointment should not be made available as an OTC particularly when it could not easily be obtained on prescription at certain times such as weekends. Anxieties were raised about the possibility of such self-medication obscuring or delaying the diagnosis of a serious underlying cause for the relatively common symptom of a painful red eye. This kind of problem is likely to be a recurring feature of any discussion directed towards the greater release of certain medicines for OTC use. What is needed in this particular example is the calculated probability of a painful red eye (in a child, a middle-aged person and the elderly) being due to either an infection or a potentially more serious problem.

More pharmacology — for the lay-person

One discussant emphasized that in devising new methods to instruct, advise and guide patients attempts to promote an understanding of elementary pharmacology should not be neglected, for example:

(1) the simple notion of a dose—response relationship;
(2) the knowledge that every drug has many effects, only one of which is likely to be the one which you are after;
(3) the likely consequences of departing from stipulated advice.

Preparation, packaging and presentation

The preparation and packaging of medicines for self-care exposed conflicting views about the use of brand names or generic drugs and the old chestnut about combined and single-drug preparations. For the first time vested and non-vested interest had entered the debate. However this is likely to be a recurring issue if, for example, it is decided to market selected preparations as packaged remedies for specific complaints and not necessarily as identifiable medicine which purchasers would be free to use in any way they chose. The advantages of this former approach include the fact that it would simplify the decisions necessary to *choose* a treatment and would avoid inappropriate actions such as the use of aspirin for dyspepsia. Approved remedies could of course be offered for common *symptom complexes;* users would not have to build their own domestic pharmacy of multiple single remedies. Experiments are needed in this area; they might be aimed at those common problems which often lead to utilization of general practice services including pain, insomnia, constipation, diarrhoea and vomiting.

On the subject of medication itself, a good example of how clear, explicit and widely agreed guidelines can be produced is the report by a multinational and multidisciplinary working group on 'Minimum information for sensible use of self-prescribed medicines' [10]. Six medicines were the subject of a coordinated analysis including nature and uses, dosage, unwanted effects and storage. The availability of such information in turn emphasizes the need to develop methods of dissemination and test their effectiveness. Recent publications concerned with the provision of explanations and advice on health and its maintenance despite a very high standard of presentation in many respects do not give any emphasis to the choice and use of home medicines [11, 12].

Whichever methods are chosen, the evaluation process must be pragmatic and will obviously be dictated by the methods used. The criteria chosen to measure effectiveness must be checked carefully. It will also be necessary to learn to tolerate an empirical approach particularly because many criteria of effectiveness are likely to be very different from those regarded as the norm by professionals.

The general conclusions of the group discussion are summaried below:

(1) Increasing attention being directed towards self-care reveals and emphasizes deficiencies in existing methods and styles of traditional medical practice.

(2) Self-care may become the most potent change-agent in educating both health personnel and the lay public about health care problems and particularly alternatives and choice.

(3) Too little is known about the subgroup within the population who would most benefit from the promotion of self-care, and those who might be disadvantaged by it.

(4) Improved opportunities for educating health personnel and the lay public must be found. Obvious opportunities exist in school programmes, in adult education and in the undergraduate and postgraduate education of health personnel concerned with primary care.

(5) Experiments based on the use of approved medicines for specified common symptom complexes provided together with explicit user guidelines (for example in the form of decision-trees) are needed, and should be carried out on defined population groups whose characteristics are properly documented.

(6) Criteria used for evaluation should be derived from users' perceptions of effectiveness and not based only on traditional concepts held by health personnel.

References

1. Levin, L. S., Katz, A. H. and Holst, E. (1976). *Self-care: Lay Initiatives in Health* (New York: Prodist)

2. Fry, J. (1975). Role of the patient in primary health care: *The Viewpoint of the Medical Practitioner.* Background paper for symposium on the role of the individual in primary care. (University of Copenhagen, Denmark: Institute of Social Medicine) (mimeographed)

3. World Health Organisation (1978). The Alma Ata Conference on Primary Health Care', *WHO Chronicle,* **32,** 409

4. *Brit. Med. J.* (leading article) 'General knowledge of cancer'. 18th November 1972, 381

5. J. M. Atkinson, personal communication

6. Zola, I. K. (1975). 'Medicine as an institution of social control'. In C. Cox and A. Meads (eds.) *A Sociology of Medical Practice.* pp. 170—185 (London: Collier-Macmillan)

7. Marsh, G. N. (1977). "Curing" minor illness in general practice. *Br. Med. J.,* **2,** 1278

8. Wilcox, B., Engel, E. and Reid, D. (1978). 'Smoking education in children: UK trials of an international project', *Int. J. Health Education,* **21,** 236

9. Essex, B. J. (1976). *Diagnostic Pathways in Clinical Medicine: An Epidemiological Approach to Clinical Problems.* (Edinburgh: Churchill Livingstone)

10. Report by an *ad hoc* working group (1977). 'Minimum information

for sensible use of self-prescribed medicines: an international consensus'. *Lancet,* **ii,** 1017

11. *Family Health Guide (1972): Reader's Digest*
12. *Odhams Home Medical Guide Cards* (London: The Hamlyn Publishing Group Limited)

5

Products for home medication

G. R. FRYERS

INTRODUCTION

In this chapter the term 'products' is used to describe not only the active ingredients included in the formulation but also the whole presentation of the preparation: that is, its immediate packaging, labelling and any information included with it.

At the outset the purposes for which home medication products are used are reviewed in order to give perspective to the problems of safety and efficacy. Consideration of the contribution a subject's 'expectation' can make to the efficacy of symptomatic products, and the implications of this fact on the methods of assessment of efficacy, lead into a brief discussion of the place of combination products in home medication.

The problems of communication on and with the pack are reviewed, together with an examination of factors that determine where and when warnings should appear. The need for communication to the medical profession to ensure that they can effectively oversee the possibility of interactions between their treatment and those taken for home medication, and between the roles of the doctor and pharmacist in advising people with special problems on the safe and effective use of home medication, is also discussed.

The chapter concludes with suggestions for a number of areas in which further research is indicated.

PURPOSES FOR WHICH HOME MEDICATION PRODUCTS MAY BE USED

(1) To treat superficial, easily recognisable conditions.

(2) To relieve the symptoms (or clusters of symptoms) of conditions which are believed to be self-limiting and, in the view of the subject, do not require medical attention. For this limited purpose an aetiological diagnosis is generally neither necessary nor achievable before taking symptomatic and general supportive measures.

(3) The supportive treatment of people with irremediable, non-life-threatening conditions who have had the benefit of medical advice and usually a diagnosis, but who have been advised by the doctor that the best course is to follow a particular regime which may include some measure of home medication.

It is useful to think of categories 1 and 2 as being the field of primary home care and category 3 as being secondary home care. The distinction is useful in that the public can initiate treatments in the primary home care field, so it is appropriate that the availability of medicines for these purposes is advertised to them. Medicines taken in the course of secondary home care should only be used on the basis of medical advice, even though a repeat prescription may not be necessary. In these circumstances the advertising of the products with their indications for use would seem to be inappropriate.

Another classification which more clearly sets the scene in regard to the totality of health care is based on the recognition of the contrast between the doctor's unique ability to make diagnoses a necessary basis for most specific treatments and the layman's restricted ability to diagnose only a few superficial conditions (those that would be included in (1) above). However, symptomatic home medication does not depend on aetiological diagnosis for its success — the field can perhaps be more accurately described as *prediagnostic medicine.*

Increasingly the doctor is concerned to make more accurate diagnoses in order to be able to use the more powerful and specific treatments that are becoming available, so that his emphasis upon diagnostic medicine will probably increase. Those patients who have been diagnosed but for whom no specific curative treatment is available, can usefully be described as being included in *postdiagnostic medicine.* If this system of classification is used then an even earlier stage than prediagnostic medicine can also be described, that of *presymptomatic medicine,* which includes conditions such as hypertension, glaucoma, diabetes, etc., which, while they exist without producing symptoms can nonetheless be recognized by special tests.

Throughout the rest of this chapter the main emphasis is on the relief of symptoms in both prediagnostic and postdiagnostic circumstances, rather than on superficial conditions which the public can learn to diagnose themselves. For the relief of symptoms a great variety of measures have been devised, some physical, some pharmaceutical; others may be psychological or even supportive devices. While it is necessary to change specific biochemical processes in order to produce a curative effect when purely symptomatic measures are the aims, the mechanism by which the efficacy is achieved is quite unimportant. The only matter of importance is the level of relief that can be achieved for an acceptable, monitored amount of risk. The several possible, acceptable inter-relationships between safety and efficacy are illustrated in Figure 5.1 below.

SOURCES OF INGREDIENTS

Because the main thrust of pharmaceutical research and development has been directed at obtaining efficacy, much less effort has gone towards

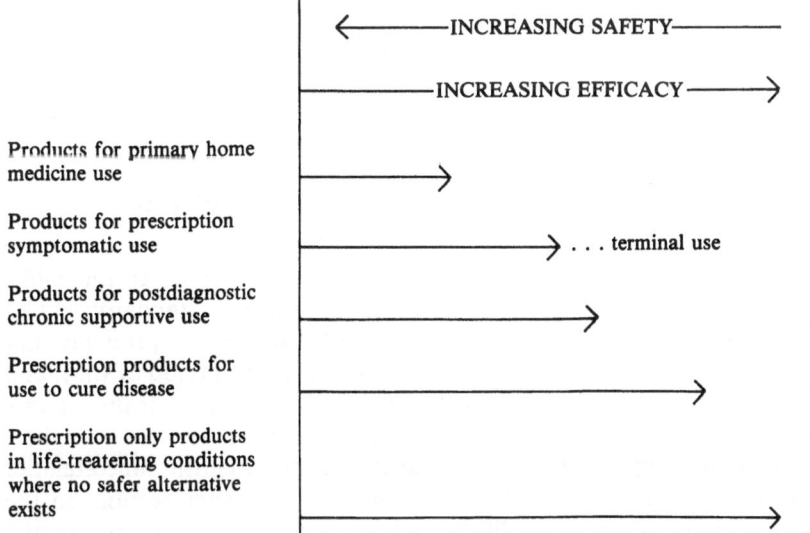

Figure 5.1 Safety and efficacy interelationships

increasing safety, though clearly efficacy has only been useful when accompanied by a reasonable level of safety. It follows that a relatively small proportion of the products introduced for prescription use will meet the exacting safety standards required for a product to be used in prediagnostic conditions. Indeed, the problems of establishing whether the characteristic safety of the product is sufficient are very hard to solve. If, for instance, it is required that a serious hazard should not occur in more than 1 in 10 000 users (who might each use the product once a week over a period of years) then we would need a study group of at least 50 000 which would be impossibly large both to recruit and to manage. Furthermore, the study would be unacceptable on ethical grounds. Consequently, we are unlikely to be able to introduce any new chemical compounds directly to the home medicine field and almost certainly not if they are for internal use. In addition there is no credible mechanism by which research and development could be organized to develop products which would first have to be used by doctors but only achieve their designed potential when they reached the home medication market; because such a process would take 15 to 20 years from inception to the successful appearance of the first home medicine, it would be impracticable to manage or finance such long-term projects.

In these circumstances the industry must expect that the only way it wil get new ingredients is by selecting the occasional product which, though designed for prescription use, proves to have an adequate record of safety. Although these 'hand-me-downs' from the prescription medicine industry must provide the input, they also need substantial amounts of further development work to make them suitable for home medication.

THE ASSESSMENT OF EFFICACY OF SYMPTOMATIC PRODUCTS

There is a large number of traditional herbal remedies which the public use for symptomatic purposes which have never been standardized and validated pharmacologically. In most of them it is probably not practicable to undertake the work, except over a long period of time, and so they may have either to be withdrawn from the market, if there is any question of their safety, or by labelling them as, for instance, 'traditional' products give an indication of scientific uncertainties surround their efficacy. As will be seen from a later section on the 'expectation effect', it is likely that many people achieve substantial benefit from these herbal products and as a result it is likely that the current review of medicines' licences will generally allow them to remain if they are labelled distinctively, in much the way that has been suggested. For symptomatic products containing ingredients that have a demonstrated pharmacological activity the standard view of medical scientists on appropriate tests of efficacy is that there should be blind, controlled studies of each formulation. This, however, is not really practicable: such studies are expensive and would contribute little or nothing to the advancement of medical science. However, it is not yet generally accepted, and little attention has so far been given to the possibility, that such a method would mislead about the effctiveness of the products under consideration and this possibility must now be examined.

In controlled studies on the relief of symptoms it has usually been shown that from 30 — 50% of subjects get very satisfactory relief from a placebo. This is often known as the placebo effect. However, this is a misnomer, in that the effect is not a property of the product but of the subject's 'expectation'. It has been shown that this 'expectation effect' can either be positive or negative. Girdwood et al. [1] showed that the placebo that resembled an active tablet in appearance produced all the same side-effects as the active tablet, whereas in the same study a placebo with other characteristics produced different effects. The greater the expectation of the subject, the greater the benefit conferred. In effect the process seems to be a reinforceable, conditioned reflex, set in motion by the subject's expectation and it is therefore better described as the 'expectation effect'.

In blind, clinical trials, the design has normally been arranged to exclude this effect. Whilst this is appropriate for determining whether a specific curative medicine achieves the results for which it was designed, it is not appropriate when the product is being presented for the relief of symptoms. The greater the contribution of the expectation effect to total benefit, the larger the therapeutic ratio ought to be. Conversely, a negative expectation which could arise from a product being offered which was similar to one that had produced a bad previous experience, will substantially detract from the favourable pharmacology that has been built-in to the product. The ideal symptomatic product can be defined as being one in which a pharmacological basis for action is supplemented by a maximal expectation effect so that the sum of these two activities produces complete symptomatic relief in a substantial number of people. If the expectation effect is to be treated as part of the active ingredient's 'effective' composition, then clearly it must not be

Table 5.1

	A 'Analgesic tablets' placebo	B Branded placebo	C 'Analgesic tablets' active	D Branded active
Mean pain relief (1 hour)	1.98	2.25	2.57	2.72
Mean pain relief (½ hour)	1.15	1.16	1.34	1.32
Complete relief at one hour	43%	50%	58%	63%

excluded from the studies of efficacy.

In a study at the University of Keele, which has not yet been published, Branthwaite and Cooper set out to test the contribution the expectation effect, associated with a widely used, branded, home medicine analgesic, contributed to the overall effectiveness of the product. They used a 2 x 2 experimental design with 869 women divided into four groups (matched as to age, social class and frequency of taking headache remedies). The four groups were each given one product. All the materials were packed in the same type of 50-tablet cannister; B and D were labelled both on the pack and on the tablet with the brand name; and A and C were labelled 'analgesic tablets' on the pack. The tablets in these packs were unlabelled but othewise of the same size and appearance as the branded products. The formulation used in products A and B contained the same placebo materials whereas C and D both used the standard active formulation of the branded product. The instructions for use were the same on all four packs. The subjects were asked to record the effect of the product with which they were supplied on any headaches they might experience in a two-week period. They scored on a six-point scale, from 'worse' to 'completely better', the degree of relief at 30 and 60 min after taking the dose (Table 5.1).

The placebo responder rates are fairly high as would be expected when people were evaluating an analgesic as opposed to a possible analgesic. That the established brand fared better than the equivalent product labelled with an unfamiliar name indicated that expectation can be built up over time and through usage. It can also be inferred that pharmacological activity added only 15% or 13% to the 43% or 50% complete relief due to the expectation effect alone.

When the subjects were asked to compare the product they had been given with their usual remedy, only the group who received the branded, active form produced better average results then they got from their usual remedy. The other groups produced less satisfactory results. These results indicate the very substantial contribution of the expectation effect to the total effectiveness of this analgesic. If the aim is, as suggested, to keep the pharmacological effect to a low, but active level and maximize the expectation effect, and if the expectation effect is going to be the larger component of efficacy in such a product, then one must question whether measurement of the pharmacology alone would contribute very much. In considering this one must also recognize the impracticability of any sort of precise measure for the symptomatic and therefore subjective variable at the lowest effective dose levels.

In all these circumstances it is concluded that once the pharmacology has been clearly demonstrated at a fuller dose, it is logical to project downwards from the proven effect to doses that are likely to be a little above the threshold of activity, and then to design a formulation and presentation such that, over time, the expectation effect will be maximized and then leave the further measurement of efficacy to the users themselves.

In the study referred to (from Keele) brands were seen to be more effective than generic presentations and, indeed, it seems likely that the expectation effect can only be built up if people believe that they are going to get the same product every time. Branding and advertising brands can, if properly conducted, contribute substantially to the build-up of the expectation effect and therefore to effectiveness and safety. The benefit achieved presumably provided the basis for the public's preference for brands. Indeed it is impossible to assess how far the effectiveness of commonly used generics such as soluble aspirin and paracetamol derives from their known close similarity to established brands of high repute.

SAFETY AND COMMUNICATION FACTORS

A high level of safety must be built into every home medicine product but even so there must always be some potential for harm. The acceptable level of risk depends on the care and understanding with which the product is used so questions of safety and communication are bound up together. Most communication must be fixed to the pack to reach the

73

user at the critical time — advertisements and leaflets may not be around when the product is used.

There are perhaps one or two uncommunicable dangers that might render a basically safe product unsuitable for home medication, for instance when it has a very long duration of action, so long that cumulation can be a serious problem. Such products seem to present insuperable difficulties, as the concept of cumulation is one which is unknown to many members of the public. It is vital that people should only use medicines according to the directions supplied with them. The risk that a few will take much larger doses or take them more frequently or for much longer periods limits the range of products that can be made available to the public as a whole. Surely, therefore, the most important, specific instructions to get across is to 'read the instructions carefully and to adhere to them'. However, people are reluctant to read and all important material must be as easily read and as compactly presented as possible. This additional information really falls into two categories:

(1) Comments that are applicable to all, or nearly, all, the users, such as injunction to 'keep the medicines out of the reach of children', or to 'consult a doctor if the symptoms persist'. Fortunately the list of these general points is quite short.

(2) The Pandora's box is opened when one considers information which might be of importance to minority groups. Here the list could be extremely long and, even if it were physically possible to supply the information, it would be overlooked if the minorities concerned did not find the material generally of importance to them. Also the very important general messages would probably be lost in the background noise. Fortunately these minority groups can only know of their problem because they have at some time obtained a medical diagnosis and this provides the key to the policy that should be adopted about such warnings. The doctor, as he does in the case of all other aspects of the regime that the patients should follow, should advise on home medicines where the patient's condition demands that special considerations apply — for instance, in the rather complex circumstances surrounding aspirin and asthma, where some may be helped and some may be made worse but most are unaffected.

However correct this policy may be in principle it may be less effective than it ought to be unless doctors take more interest in home medication. They rarely ask their patients for a history of self-treatment and may therefore overlook the importance of giving advice, even though it is appropriate. Doctors ought to be an important source of advice and information on home medication.

Pregnancy deserves some special comment, although a minority subject numerically (at any one time about 0.3 of the United Kingdom population will be pregnant). Pregnancy is generally only confirmed after a visit to a doctor. A general caution about medicines and pregnancy would cause confusion because any woman of fertile age who had had intercourse might in fact be pregnant. If all were to be cautioned not to take any pharmaceutical preparation without their doctor's agreement, he would have to advise almost all women in this age group — surely an unreal and unconstructive proposal, particularly if we are talking about medicine being used in dosages where studies so far have failed to show any harm to either mother or baby. Perhaps it would be more logical to forbid products from the home medicine field where a pregnancy risk was established and at the same time to maintain the current position that there should be no pregnancy warnings on labels of the surviving products.

COMBINATION PRODUCTS

In the case of the common cold, and a number of other conditions, symptoms do not come individually but in clusters. There are then the possible alternatives of treating by a separate product for each symptom, or by a fixed dose of a combination product for all of them at one time. The duration of these symptoms is often only a day or two; titration of dosage is impracticable and the knowledge required in order to use several medicines simultaneously is unlikely ever to be present in the general population. For all of these reasons fixed-dose combination products have an important place in the treatment of clusters of symptoms which occur in relatively predictable patterns. Their efficacy must be determined by logical extrapolation, much in the same way as that for single-ingredient home medicines, and again the maximum 'expectation effect' should be built-in to the presentation, the pack, and its promotion, subject always to the promotion being honest and truthful.

If a person finds a particular medicine to be making claims beyond his limits of credulity, then it seems likely that he/she will approach its use with some suspicion and a negative expectation effect will be built in. It may have been some unverbalized understanding of the vital need for credibility that led the home medicine industry in the UK to be the first industry in the world to impose on its members a voluntary promotional code, to bring credible order from the earlier state in which unjustified and excessive promotional claims were prevalent.

PRODUCTS FOR PRIMARY DIAGNOSTIC HOME MEDICATION

These are for use where the public can make a diagnosis such as warts, corns, mouth ulcers, burns, scalds, insect bites, and acne. The conditions are relatively few, and they are all superficial, and for them to be suitable for home medication they must be ones that the public can easily learn to recognize. Here the remedies can be curative and the standards of efficacy should be those that generally apply to other curative medicine. There do not appear to be any special problems about communication or safety for this category of product.

POSTDIAGNOSTIC OR SECONDARY HOME MEDICATION

This field is one which has been quite inadequately researched. Very little is known about it. The archetypal condition is, say, an older man with an osteoarthritic knee who has relapses from time to time; he may need to take aspirin in larger doses and for a longer period than would be appropriate for prediagnostic home medication. Clearly it is important that the dosage instructions on the label should permit only the dose that he is recommended to use by his doctor. Indeed, if there is no product with a label indicating the necessary dose level then either the doctor must continue to prescribe so that special labels are written, or the pharmacist will provide a suitable label, or some other change must be made, because over a long period of time memory is fallible, the dosage might be confused and serious danger arise.

As stated earlier, the indications in this category of home medication seem not to be suitable for advertising but if safety is to be maintained the instructions that go with the product must be extremely clear.

THE NEED FOR ADDITIONAL PRODUCTS

In the field of prediagnostic medicine there are a number of conditions for which no home medicine is offered. This is usually because the available effective ingredients have not been proven to have sufficient safety; occasionally it appears to be due to *conservatism*. A possible example of the latter is to be found in the short-term treatment of local skin conditions; for instance, 0.5% hydrocortisone is prescribed frequently without the aetiology being clear. The fears of adverse effects stem from experience of widespread and long-term usage. Should not 0.5% hydrocortisone products be available as a home medication for the temporary relief of local skin conditions?

The need for a sedative is also fairly clear but here the problem is whether any ingredient is sufficiently free of the tendency to product dependence on it. Whether any of the nitrazepam—diazepam family, or the sedative antihistamines could be used with safety has not yet been established. Perhaps a 'pharmacy only' product, with all sales recorded and limited to small-sized packs, would provide sufficient assurances against misuse, whilst allowing the necessary experience to be accumulated.

There are at present more questions than answers. It is, however, a measure of progress that the subject of self-medication has been defined to the point where it is now possible to frame some pertinent questions.

References

1. Moertel, C. G., Taylor, W. F., Roth, A. and Tyce, F. A. J. (1976). Who responds to sugar pills? *Mayo Clin. Proc.*, **51**, 96
2. Girdwood, R. D. (1976). Personal communication

Supplementary discussion — points for consideration

Supplementary discussion — points for consideration

(1) What are the limits to, and the quantitive scale of, the field of secondary home medication?

(2) What is the contribution of the 'expectation effect' in symptomatic home medication?

(3) What is the role of the community pharmacist in:

    (a) advising new users of home medicines?

    (b) advising on changes in usage?

    (c) advising on choice of preparation to comply with medical recommendations on secondary home medication?

(4) How best can important instructions be conveyed to users?

    (a) on and with packs?

    (b) by pharmacists?

    (c) by doctors?

(5) How much information can be communicated effectively? And what are the priorities if the amount is limited?

(6) Many people consult doctors for conditions which others would generally effectively look after themselves. Why do they do so? How far is it due to lack of products or awareness of products?

(7) How do patients cope when they have chronic low-grade conditions which doctors fail to recognize and treat? Do such people misuse home medication?

(8) What additional symptoms or conditions are suitable for primary home medication? Are there suitable ingredients that might be used?

Supplementary discussion

Chairman: J. Crooks
Prime discussant: J. E. Iles
Rapporteur: P. N. Bennett

The group considered the following questions:

(1) *What are the limits to, and the quantitive scale of, the field of secondary home medication?*

'Secondary home medication' is the use of non-prescribed drugs by patients for irremediable but non-life-threatening conditions. It thus refers to particular classes of medication likely to be used recurrently rather than to the whole range of symptomatic remedies. Definition of the scale of this type of medication and the identification of potential benefits and hazards could help to clarify the role of self-medication in health care in general. A patient's decision to treat himself can be regarded as a potential saving to the NHS in tems of prescribing cost or manpower if few visits are made to the doctor. On the other hand, the limits to secondary medication are probably defined either by the potential for toxicity of the drugs used or by the danger of preventable deterioration in the underlying disease if the patient is not reviewed periodically by his doctor. Analgesic nephropathy and subacute myelo-optic neuropathy (SMON) from treatment with clioquinol are recent reminders that home medicines can cause serious harm to patients. Another potential problem is that doctors may not be aware that their patients are self-medicating. For example, clinical trials to establish whether aspirin or aspirin-like drugs reduce the incidence of myocardial infarction are in progress. A premature impression that such drugs are protective may induce patients with ischaemic heart disease to take aspirin prophylactically and this may lead to renal damage or gut bleeding.

The issue of self-medication is worth considering because it explores the interface between prescribed and non-prescribed medicines. Examination of the problem may show that the availability of some medicines for instance some antihistamines is unnecessarily restrictive; by the same token, unwanted effects of seemingly innocuous medicines may come to light. Drug surveillance programmes have identified adverse reactions to a number of prescribed medicines and such work is aided by the fact that both the drugs and the patients taking them are known. By contrast the problems of detecting harmful effects in sporadically taken home medicines must be greater. Nevertheless in relation to secondary home medication the exercise seems worth attempting since the patients can be identified as those with chronic or recurrent illnesses for which home medicines can offer relief, for example chronic joint disorders, dyspepsia or dysmenorrhoea. An investigation into the proper scope of secondary home medication could well concentrate on these areas.

(2) *What is the contribution of the 'expectation effect' in symptomatic home medication?*

The expectation effect and the pharmacological effect both contribute to the patient's overall response to therapy and both can be an undesirable as well as a desirable experience. All doctors are aware that patients can have side-effects to one brand but not to another of what is in fact the same compound. Tablet colour has also been known to affect response to treatment. It is recognized that doctors can themselves generate an expectation effect by the degree of enthusiasm with which they advocate particular medicines to their patients; indeed this can be a positive part of therapy. Likewise the drug industry seeks to create an expectation of benefit from its products — indeed this is one objective of advertising.

In relation to home medicines there are several reasons why an expectation effect might contribute to the total therapeutic effect beyond that achieved by a drug's pharmacological action. Firstly the effects of most of these agents are relatively mild; secondly they are bought on the patient's own initiative and with his own money; thirdly the benefits which may be expected to result from their use may be widely proclaimed in the advertising media. These factors will have to be acknowledged in any attempt to study the use of home medicines in a systematic way, as in clinical trials. Indeed the mechanisms, magnitude and role of the expectation effect in home medicines is itself worthy of investigation.

(3) *What is the role of the community pharmacist in:*
   (a) *advising new users of home medicines?*
   (b) *advising on changes in usage?*
   (c) *advising on choice of preparation to comply with medical recommendations on secondary home medication?*

The community pharmacist is clearly well-placed to advise users of home medicines in that he is physically accessible for patients with minor ailments requiring symptomatic relief — conditions which may largely have cleared by the time an appointment can be obtained with the general practitioner. The pharmacist's knowledge of the range of home medicines and of the detail of their constituents is extensive and he is thus an appropriate person to advise on their use. An important proviso is that the information should come from the pharmacist and not from other shop staff. In one survey [1], it was found that information on health care obtained from pharmacists was thought by members of the public to be useful. Indeed advising on the symptomatic relief of minor conditions has been part of the traditional role of the pharmacist. The limitation of that role is lack of training which pharmacists receive in the nature of disease processes and this deficiency is recognized in that most schools of pharmacy now include courses in clinical medicine in their curricula. Clearly there is advantage to be gained if the pharmacist can interpret the possible significance of a recurrent symptom, such as persistant cough being due to a lung neoplasm; or 'indigestion' being due to angina. Utilizing the pharmacist in what is in fact an extension of the accepted role, that is, to play a part in early diagnosis, could be good preventive medicine. To this end it would be valuable to know to what extent the average retail pharmacist appreciates the significance of selected important signs and symptoms. This could readily be assessed by standard methods like a questionnaire. A programme in which community pharmacists were positively encouraged to question customers about the symptoms for which they are seeking remedies may well reveal treatable disease. The value of such an exercise should be assessed.

(4) *How best can important instructions be conveyed to users?*
   (a) *on and with packs?*
   (b) *by pharmacists?*
   (c) *by doctors?*

Package inserts can carry quite a lot of detailed information but the more that is given the less is the patient likely to read it. Instructions on packs are less likely to get lost but simply because of physical limitation in size the information on them is best confined to the most important points. Nevertheless compliance with the taking of home medicines is aided by the fact that many are used for only short periods for symptomatic relief. Indeed adherence to instructions is probably better than that for prescribed medicines.

Clearly the pharmacist who is present at the sale of home medicines is in an excellent position to advise on their use and to caution about adverse effects. Indeed the level of understanding of potential dangers of non-prescribed medicines in the general public is in its own right a subject worth exploring. It would also be valuable to establish in what proportions of sales of home medicines advice as to their use is currently either sought or given. A logical extension of this notion would be to investigate whether routine verbal instruction of customers by pharmacists at the time of sale is an effective means of communicating information. Studies such as these, none of which would appear to present insurmountable difficulty, could show whether this mechanism of health education, that is via the dispensing pharmacist, is of real value, and if so whether it is being optimally utilized.

The doctor from a position of having a knowledge of both the patient's disease and of other drugs he may be taking should be an important source of advice. However he may be unaware that his patients are self-medicating. Indeed patients may not volunteer the information since they frequently do not regard medicines which they buy in supermarkets, such as aspirin or paracetamol, as being drugs. Probably doctors should be more attuned to eliciting from patients whether they are taking home medicines. It should be part of medical student training that in taking a drug history, questions about non-prescribed medicines should be asked.

The potential role of the nurse in communicating to patients about home medicines, and indeed about drugs in general has been neglected. Yet nurses, either in attachment to general practices or as health visitors, are readily accessible to patients and by clinical training and experience they are well-placed to advise about home medicines. The value of the nurse in this role should be explored and developed.

(5) *How much information can be communicated effectively? What are the priorities if the amount is limited?*

Both the quantity of information and the manner in which it is presented are important. If the data presented is too bulky the patient will not read it all; the amount of information given must be a matter of judgement for individual medicines. Obviously dosage and any modification for age should be clearly stated; so also should any precautions particular to the drug under consideration, for instance, unexpected drowsiness due to alcohol with preparations containing an antihistamine. Attention to the design of package inserts or container labels could help to highlight important pieces of information. Consideration could be given to the use of symbols of diagrams rather than to script to make important points. It would be of interest to test, for selected products, whether members of the general public do actually read accompanying instructions and precautions and whether they remember and act on them.

(6) *How do patients cope when they have chronic low-grade conditions which doctors fail to recognize and treat? Do such people misuse home medication?*

A proportion of patients who, for whatever reason, feel dissatisfied with prescribed medicines may well turn to over-the-counter preparations. Self-medication may indeed be a way in which they can obtain symptomatic relief, but in some of these patients there must be a danger that excessive delay in coming to a diagnosis may lead to permanent harm, or that chronic self-medication leads to adverse effects, for example the chronic use of cathartics may permanently damage bowel motility. The problem of trying to establish whether a significant proportion of self-medicators come to harm is partly that of identifying the population. A reasonable starting point might be to examine attenders with complaints such as backache, dysmenorrhoea or bowel dysfunction for evidence of drug misuse.

(7) *What additional symptoms or conditions are suitable for primary home medication? Are there suitable ingredients that might be used?*

In one sense these questions relate to the boundary between the drugs which are prescribed by a doctor and those which he can obtain for himself. There are certain areas in which this might be explored, for example, a limited availability of diuretics for premenstrual fluid retention or, possibly, steroid-containing applications for certain skin conditions. One approach might be to make available selected drugs on a 'pharmacy only' basis — in other words, these drugs could be obtained on a pharmacist's signature provided arrangements are made for the patient to be reviewed at stipulated intervals by a doctor. Since such a system would represent a departure from current practice its advantages would need to be clearly demonstrable before it could be generally accepted.

Reference

1. Elliot-Binns (1973). An analysis of lay medicine. *J. R. Coll. Gen. Practit.*, **23**, 255

6

Relations with health care professions and public

J. FRY

SELF-CARE

Among the priorities for better health over the next 25 years, the concept of self-care must be high on the list for actions and benefits.

We have reached a stage in medical history when the limitations of technological and professional medical care are apparent and when a reorientation is necessary.

The cost of medical technology has escalated to frightening levels and the cost-benefits for better health, disease control and prevention are such that enormous amounts of money and manpower are increasingly required to achieve small improvements. More and more money is being spent for less and less improvements in personal and public health.

Health care and health are essentially about the health of the people and about health of the individual and his family. Health care should be more about how individuals can become healthy and stay healthy and how they might avoid diseases, accidents and premature death, than about how the NHS or other medical and social services should be organized, reorganized and re-reorganized, or what should be the interprofession and intraprofessional demarcation lines among doctors, nurses and social workers.

Within the complex issues of providing health care making the services available, accessible, affordable, adaptable, assessible and acceptable, the place of self-care and the individual's own responsibilities for his or her own health are all important. Until recently it has been relatively neglected as a potent force to better health.

SELF-RESPONSIBILITIES

A review of our health indices over the past 25 years will show that there have been *no reductions in the extent of morbidity* as evidenced by the rates of consultations in general practice, by use of hospital outpatient, inpatient, accident, and emergency and diagnostic services. Life-expectancy for middle aged men and women has scarcely improved. We have sunk lower in the health league as measured by infant mortality. Sickness absence is increasing and so is the prescribing of drugs by general practitioners.

The use of health services is intimately related to personal habits and mores and to prevailing social conditions, lifestyles and public expectations and demands, and to national morale, frustrations, restrictions, shortages and inflation.

It is likely that we tend to overuse, misuse and abuse our health services. There is a general assumption that there has to be a free and freely available naitonal health service in which must exist the principles of full professional clinical freedom for doctors to order and prescribe what they think right.

It is almost too late because the NHS is more or less bankrupt. There may still be a chance to slow down our headlong rush for more and more and more medical resources by considering some of our own *self-responsibilities* for health and health care.

These responsibilities must apply to health care professionals as well as to the public. There has to be a public debate on what is useful and what is useless in health care. There will have to be a more realistic and a more commonsensical approach to health care, to health promotion, health maintenance, disease prevention and disease control.

One of the best prospects for better health is the individual's responsibilities for his own health. *Much of the prevailing poor health in our society is caused by personal bad habits.* The rules of good health are well known, and unexciting — stop smoking, eat less, drink less, take regular exercise, avoid stress and get enough sleep. There is nothing new in these rules — every schoolboy and schoolgirl knows them. But departure from them has led to the current pandemics of cancer of the lung, ischaemic heart diseases, obesity and mental illness.

The challenge to better health in the immediate future is: *how can we motivate the individual to change his (or her) bad personal habits for the better?*

THE WIDER IMPLICATIONS OF SELF-CARE

There is much more to self-care than self-medication. Some tend to equate self-care with caring for one-self with over-the-counter-remedies for minor illnesses and not bothering the doctor. Self-medication is a very small part of self-care, although a necessary part. Self-care includes self-care for minor illnesses but more importantly it must include measures for health maintenance and disease prevention. It must include close cooperation with the medical profession and health services in care and prevention. It must include knowledge of how best to use available health services.

Who does what?

We all have responsibilities. We must all be involved in the challenge to motivate ourselves and the public to better self-care. We all have roles. We cannot and must not leave it to the Health Education Council, to the DHSS, to the public health workers, to the hospitals, to the general practitioner, or to others. We must all act as a single greater medical profession and accept the challenges.

One purpose of this Workshop is to define the needs of better self-care and the roles of us all in it.

THE PUBLIC

I have great respect for the public. I believe that the great majority of individuals in our society are anxious to do what they can to get healthy and to keep healthy, and are prepared to become involved in self-care and in self-help health measures. I believe that the great majority are anxious to collaborate with health care professionals and to use available services with care and discrimination.

I think the public has been less than well provided with sound and reliable information, facts and education on health matters. They have been fed on newsworthy and sensational medical miracles by the media.

It is necessary to emphasize more the limitations of modern medicine, to spell out what it can and what it cannot do. We need to agree on a policy of re-education of the public on the realities of health and disease and on the roles and responsibilities of self-care. We need to consider what might be done, how it might be done, who might do it, where, when and how the effects might be measured and monitored.

THE MEDICAL PROFESSION

As a profession we have been obsessed by the 'Acting-like-God' (or 'ALG' syndrome, assuming that the only important matters in health and health care are what *we* do. As a profession we will have to accept the public, our patients, as intelligent and helpful collaborators and colleagues in the whole process of health and health care. We need as a profession re-education and reorientation to help us to form a better relationship with the public, and re-education must involve all levels from the undergraduate stage up to established senior practitioners.

Each contact and consultation with our patients should involve some consideration of the part that self-care may contribute to the patients' health.

PRIMARY CARE TEAM

The first contact and long-term continuing care that the primary care team provides to a relatively small and well-known community offers very special opportunities to promote the principles of better self-care.

The general practitioner is but one member of this team — by no means the most important one. Often forgotten are the medical secretaries and receptionsits of the practice who provide the real first contact with patients, and give information on common medical and health problems. Many have had little training for their work and certainly none on how to promote and to encourage better self-care.

The nurses and health visitors attached to the practice are undertaking more structured health care in primary care. They have very special opportunities to promote self-care in their visits to homes and in health centres and practice premises.

The general practitioner in the NHS should have special incentives to encourage his patients to better self-care. Such care will reduce unnecessary work for him as well as promote better health. The whole primary care team, in fact should become involved in a more structured approach to self-care. This will require re-education of primary care team on principles of self-care and on effective methods of promoting it in their own practice communities. Such a re-education process will need a curriculum, a system and a drive to promote it nationally and locally at postgraduate centres and through medical news media.

THE PHARMACIST

Relations between pharmacists and general practice have tended to be remote and unconstructive. The pharmacist, however, is involved in much self-care. He acts as adviser on common problems. He sells over-the-counter preparations that at any time some -60% of the population is using; of this, 30% are taking some prescribed drugs and 30% are using some self-medication products supplied by pharmacists. The pharmacist must be brought into structured health care programmes and must collaborate more closely with his medical colleagues.

A few pioneering collaborative trials have started. There is a great need to support research projects to see how better relationships can be established between pharmacists and medical services.

OTHER COMMUNITY HEALTH AREAS

Social workers, voluntary workers and many others are involved in local health care providing help and advice. They must be included in any schemes to encourage and promote better self-care, so in planning, consideration must be given to such workers in self-care promotion.

District hospitals exercise important effects on health care policy. District hospital consultants, nurses and administrations must become involved and active in self-care promotion, and be included in local efforts.

NATIONAL BODIES

Self-care must be accepted as an important priority for better health. A national programme and a national body should be created to promote this. A national organization (possibly the Health Education Council) should take the first step and convene a group to agree on such a step.

Any national body for self-care promotion should accept the fact that most of the effective work will be carried out in the community. Its main efforts should be to provide the stimulus, incentives and the resources by which the work can be done.

Supplementary discussion — points for consideration

(1) What is the case for self-care with particular reference to home medication.

(2) What should be the roles and the responsibilities in self-care for:

    (a) the public?
    (b) the individual and the family?
    (c) the primary care team?
    (d) the pharmacist?
    (e) the community health workers?
    (f) the district hospital?
    (g) national bodies?

(3) How can self-care be promoted and what should be the first steps?

(4) Should there be a national policy?

(5) What contribution can be made by activities at local level to improve self-care?

Supplementary discussion

Chairman: J. H. Walker
Prime discussants: S. Currey and J. Davis
Rapporteur: P. A. Parish

The group accepted that the appropriate and safe use of effective and safe medicinal products is an important part of self-care. If such use is to improve then the individual who seeks relief from symptoms will require educating about which disorders to self-treat, the selection of appropriate medicines and when to seek medical advice. However the questions posed by Fry were deemed to be so inter-related that it would be more profitable to discuss their general implication than to try and answer the questions individually.

Members of the primary health care team have an important role and responsibility in the community to encourage individuals to take on such responsibility for their own health maintenance. But if this responsibility is to be encouraged and developed then the primary health care team needs to become a reality. At present it remains but an ideology. Because of differing views about health care and a lack of understanding between each professional about the other's knowledge and skills the contribution which the primary health care team could make in the community has seldom been realized. Conflict rather than cooperation has often developed and the need for groups of health care workers to protect their professional boundaries has often been given priority over the needs of the patient who seeks relief from pain and suffering.

Protection of professional boundaries has also acted as a barrier to the dissemination of information among health care professionals. Yet in the area of medicinal therapies a major deficiency exists between knowledge which is available about medicines and its application to the treatment of patients. Other deficiencies include the education of doctors, nurses and particularly patients about medicines and their appropriate and safe use. The health service is structured around individualized services and the doctor legitimates his role in terms of the need to individualize and particularize treatment in an individual patient — this is called clinical judgement. Such an approach requires that the doctor has special knowledge of the patient, the disorder to be treated and the medicines to be used. This not only requires knowledge, but also skill and experience, and with the rapid advances in therapeutics it must be asked whether it is realistic to expect a family doctor to keep up to date with advances in medical knowledge as well as advances in clinical pharmacology and therapeutics. Such expectations are unreal, and in future the inclusion of the pharmacist in the health care team, with his unique knowledge of medicines, could help to complement the role of the family doctor in improving health care. The pharmacist's education will need restructuring to become more patient-focused, and the commercial pressures on the pharmacist will have to be lessened if he is to provide a more professional service and educative role.

The need for health care professionals and patients to educate each other must be recognized and the development of patient committees and self-help groups should be encouraged. Much of the doctor's time is spent in treating self-limiting diseases, and the encouragement of patients to accept responsibility for self-care of these disorders could lead to a reduction in the workload on general practitioners leaving them more time for special groups of patients. In the area of medicinal therapies the need for different levels of knowledge among health care professionals and patients must be recognized. Among non-medically qualified personnel and patients there is also a need to develop a triage system of when and when not to treat without medical advice.

Many of the deficiencies in the appropriate and safe use of medicines stem from poor communications between health care professionals and between health care professionals and patients. Education is a sociological process and depends upon good communications which depends upon good relationships. These are often determined by attitudes and expectations which are the consequence of past experiences and contemporary influences — patients live their illnesses socially. The social context in which medicines are prescribed and used should always be considered when discussing future plans to encourage self-care and the appropriate and safe use of medicines.

The general conclusion of the group was that there was need for research into the roles and responsibilities of the various health care professionals, into methods of improving the dissemination of information and into ways of improving communications.

In encouraging self-care, self-medication should not be seen as providing solutions to all health problems. Alternatives to medicinal treatments should be considered, the limitations of treatment medicine should be emphasized, and the seeking of an asymptomatic state of health should be projected as an unnecessary and unrealistic goal.

The following additional references were felt to be relevant to the theme of the discussion and its conclusion:

Royal College of General Practitioners (1967). Family health care: the team. RCGP

Wise, H. *et al.* (1976). *Making Health Teams Work.* (Ballinger)

Rabkin, M. T. (1976). Bringing the individuals together to form a team. *Bull. N. Y. Acad. Med.,* (1976). **52,** 1148

Kindig, D. A. (1975). Interdisciplinary education for primary health care team delivery. *J. Med. Educ.,* **50,** 97

Parish, P. A. (1977). Integration of academic curricula in health care. In: Van der Kleijn, E. (ed.). *Clinical Pharmacy.* (Amsterdam: Elsevier), pp. 157

Parish, P. A. (1976). Medicinal treatments: the future role of the physician and pharmacist'. *Pharm. I.,* **217,** 241

Fletcher, C. M. (1973). *Communication in Medicine.* (Nuffield Provincial Hospitals Trust

7

Self-medication in the context of self-care: a review

J. McEWEN

INTRODUCTION

Self-medication is probably one of the most important aspects of self-care as well as being one of the easiest to examine. However, it is not something separate from the wider field of self-care and its intimate relationship with the other activities must be recognized. Self-care is part of the overall process of coping with problems related to health. It may involve discussion with family, friends and relevant members of the community and reliance on them for support and help. Also it cannot be separated from the direct contact with the various sources of professional care and advice. Equally, it is related to recognized ways of dealing with a much wider range of issues by the individual and community, the cultural social and religious values of that community and the structure of society.

Self-medication appears to take three main forms:
 (1) The use of substances considered to maintain or promote health or prevent illness.
 (2) Treatment of self-limiting conditions or the early ill-defined stages of more serious illness. This is usually designed primarily to relieve symptoms, but may also be considered to be curative.
 (3) Treatment taken in addition to professionally prescribed care and medication in more serious illness or chronic conditions.

In all three aspects, there are other factors which may help achieve the desired aim — alteration in diet, more or less exercise, taking a rest, having a holiday, reduction in work, warmth, fresh air, bread poultices and so on. Self-medication must be seen in the context of self care.

Although this chapter is primarily concerned with the use of medicines, it must be remembered that alcohol and other substances may be used to achieve some of the same purposes — Some aspects of the normal use of medicines may be very similar to the normal use of alcohol [1] — the gin and tonic for relaxation after a hard day at the office, the nightcap to encourage sleep, and the glass of tonic wine for the person feeling a 'little run down'.

NORMALITY OF SYMPTOMS AND ILLNESS EXPERIENCE

Feeling unwell is a common experience although this has often been expressed in various ways. This has been clearly demonstrated over many years in community studies in different countries [2—5]: the Peckham Experiment [6], carried out prior to the Second World War provides a classical example.

At first sight, it would appear that there is a contradiction between peoples' estimate of their state of health and expressed health complaints. Wadsworth and his colleagues [2], when they asked their study population the question, 'would you say that your state of health, during the last fourteen days was perfect, good, fair or poor?', found that, although respondents assessed their state of health as perfect — 35%, good — 34%, fair — 20% and poor — 10%, in only 4.9% were no health complaints reported. This clearly indicates that symptoms are regarded as normal and compatible with 'good' or even 'perfect' health. Other studies all confirm the normality of symptoms and illness experience although results vary depending on the techniques used to gather information and the population studied. The keeping of a health diary [7] usually produces a record of more frequent symptom experience. In general higher rates have been described in new towns [8—12], certain types of housing [12—14], among young women [7, 12, 13, 15], and those who consider their health to be poor [3]. Dunnell and Cartwright [3] sum up the situation by stating that the majority of the population report at least one symptom during a 2-week period.

The cumulative experience of an individual has also been investigated [16]. One American study [17] found that during a 20-year period, the average lower-middle class male, between 20 and 45 years, experienced approximately one life-endangering illness, 20 disabling illnesses, 200 non-disabling illnesses and 1000 symptomatic episodes — one new episode every six days. By taking account of the family or household, it is suggested that the average family experiences and copes with illness on one day in four [18, 19]. If chronic illness in older family members is found in approximately half the families [20], the overall experience of coping with symptoms and illness in the family context is extremely widespread.

Studies which have examined how this burden of illness and symptoms is coped with have clearly indicated that initially and in most cases completely, this is done by the individual, the family and the community. Few reach the general practitioner and fewer reach the hospital [2—4, 21—24]. Morell and Wale [7] found that only one in 37 of the symptoms were taken to the doctor and that patients were highly selective in deciding which symptoms are appropriate for medical care.

Most of the symptoms are general or rather vague. Bell and her colleagues [12, 13], in a study in a Scottish new town, reported the following breakdown:

Tiredness, feeling run down	60%
Headaches	49%
Backache	29%
Colds	27%
Coughs	24%
Skin trouble	20%

Relating complaints to disease classification, Wadsworth and his colleagues [2] found the commonest system affected was the respiratory system, followed by mental and psychoneurotic disorders, and the bones and organs of movement.

Self-medication would seem to be the normal way of coping with problems, primarily of a symptomatic nature in the community. Is this the result of longstanding tradition and experience showing that self-medication is effective, or is it because the professional care system will not or cannot cope?

MEDICATION
Availabiliity

Most studies that have examined the subject have compared and contrasted prescribed and non-prescribed medication [2, 3, 12, 13, 21].

These studies have generally shown a greater proportion of non-prescribed medicines, both kept in the home and used by individuals.

The stocks of medicine held in a house, and the purchasing of over-the-counter medicines provides a useful indicator of a family's preparedness for coping with illness as well as reflecting its previous experience. Dunnell and Cartwright [3] in Britain found an average of 7.3 non-prescription and 3.0 prescription medicines in a household, while higher figures of 17.2 non-prescription and 5.3 prescription medicines were recorded in the United States [19] — the latter studies consistently record frequent purchasing of over-the-counter medicines [20]. In Britain, most households have immediate access to some home medicines, 91% having one or more medicines [3, 25]. Nearly all have analgesics and skin cream, one-fifth had sedatives, tranquillisers or sleeping pills and two-fifths had one or more items that the informant could not identify. (This last would indicate a potentially hazardous situation with regard to future consumption.)

Self-care for minor injury is a slightly different aspect and a survey [26] in the United States found that 98% of houses kept the basic elements for treating minor injuries — bandages, adhesive plaster, gauze and cotton-wool.

Consumption

Approximately twice as much use of non-prescribed as prescribed medicines appears to be the general finding in Britain and this seems to have remained fairly constant during the last 20 years [2, 3, 12, 13, 21]. An exception to this is reported in the study by Hannay [27] in Glasgow, who found nearly equal numbers of adults, one-third of the population, taking both prescribed and non-prescribed substances.

In an extensive international study, Kohn and White [5] found the highest rates of medication in the United States of America and Canada, where up to 75% of the populations studied were on medication — 40% being self-medication. The lowest rates were recorded in Poland and Yugoslavia with 28% on medication — 10% being self-medication. They reported considerable stability of patterns within countries and in general found that medication increased with age and was higher for females than males.

In summary, they concluded that,

'in most study areas there is substantial self-medication and even use of medicines whose contribution to health seems doubtful at best. Overall use of medicines tends to be high, perhaps even disproportionate, in relationship to levels of perceived morbidity and chronicity, and there is the suggestion that consumption of at least non-prescribed medicines may be directly related to economic descriptors of relative financial affluence.

Nature of medication

Although, generally self-medication by non-prescribed medicines is the definitive approach in the majority of episodes — up to 68% [19] — there is a combined approach of prescribed and non-prescribed medicines found in a sizeable minority of cases [3].

Medication is frequently multiple [3, 20], possibly related to the fact that symptoms are frequently multiple, and approximately half of those who self-medicate take more than one medicine. This is complicated further, since, many over-the-counter preparations are themselves composed of several substances. Bell [12, 13] reported that the 80% on medication consisted of: 40% taking one medication; 39% between two and five medicines, and 1% more than five types of medicine.

The largest single category of over-the-counter products, accounting for 50% of the self-medication is analgesics and antipyretics [2, 3, 12, 13, 20]. (In some studies these are combined, in others they are separated.) This is followed in decreasing order by cough medicines, skin preparations, indigestion mixtures, and tonics and vitamins. Although aspirin and painkillers were the commonest preparations in adults, skin ointments and antiseptics were the commonest in children [3] — reflecting the varying symptom patterns in adults and children and possibly the differing perceptions of which complaints it is appropriate to take to professional care. Many self-prescribed medicines are taken over a prolonged period [3]. More than half the items of self-prescribed analgesics and laxatives taken by adults were well-tried remedies that had first been used more than 10 years before the study interview.

In a study of a small self-contained community, Jones [28] was able to gain additional information on self-medication by simultaneous recording of doctor—patient contacts and chemist sales. This confirmed other studies that twice as many people went to the chemist to buy their own medicines as consulted the doctor, but there were variations with the different symptom complexes examined. People were more content to treat their own symptoms of coughs, colds and indigestion than they were to treat symptoms of sickness and diarrhoea. The number of people asking the chemist's advice before buying was much higher than reported in other studies and may reflect the high esteem which the chemist had in that particular community.

Few studies have described in detail the contribution of traditional or home remedies. Elliott-Binns [29] found that home remedies (those which traditionally come from the kitchen, household or garden) accounted for 15% of all advice given by the lay system. Female relatives advised them more frequently than male relatives, while the widowed and separated used them more often than the married. They were recommended progressively more frequently by the older age groups, except that teenagers advised them more often than expected. The acceptance rate for home remedies was less than for over-the-counter medicines. Bell [12, 13] found little use of traditional remedies, but this may be related to the specific social characteristics and lack of social networks in a new town. According to the Herbal Society [30], there is an increasing use of old and new herbal remedies.

The main emphasis has been on medication designed to relieve symptoms or to attempt cure of a condition. Studies in the Untied States and Britain have indicated an increasing interest in health-promoting activities, although much of this cannot be described as self-medication. Medicines designed to promote health or prevent illness were consumed on about 30% of all adult days and 25% of child-days, with vitamin preparations being commonly used [21, 31, 32]. This is very closely related to the belief that 'good' food is most important for health and that a major cause of ill-health is poor, inadequate or improper food [33].

THREE SPECIAL EXAMPLES OF DECISION-MAKING RELATED TO MEDICATION
Those who do nothing

It is interesting to comment briefly on this group. Wadsworth and his colleagues [2] reported that no action was taken by 18.8% of respondents with health problems. While some of this may be accounted for by acute, very shortlived conditions, Bell [12, 13] found that for certain chronic conditions no action might also be taken; 50% of those who felt run down and 81% of those with backache did nothing. While it is only possible to speculate as to the reasons, it may be that these conditions are accepted as a 'part of life'. As Festinger [34] has pointed out, when people believe that they cannot change a situation, they often come to believe that it is satisfactory, because it is the only way that they can get rid of the sense of unease and worry arising from the wish to change something that they think is unchangeable.

Alteration in prescribed medication

A review [35] of 68 studies of patient compliance with doctors' advice showed that an average of 44% of patients did not follow the advice given to them. This may range from not taking the prescribed medicine at all, through altering the dosage or duration, to keeping some of the prescribed medication for future use, or even giving it to someone else. Dunnell and Cartwright [3] summarize the position as: 2.5% of prescriptions are not filled at all; 16% are thrown away before being used up; and 20% are not taken as advised.

Alteration of dosage or cessation of treatment before the prescribed course is completed is usually labelled as non-compliance [36], but may indicate purposeful cessation. This may be the result of side-effects (perhaps not adequately explained at the consultation when the treatment was prescribed) or rapid improvement in the condition (the necessity of completing a course of antibiotics even if the patient feels better may not have been fully explained or understood) or the patient may be following the advice of those in his lay-referral system (family, friends or colleagues who consider the treatment inappropriate or dangerous and advise him not to follow the professional advice).

The Repeat Prescription

The continuation of medication by means of the repeat prescription, in certain instances is the antithesis of non-compliance. Here the patient decides either with or without contacting the doctor that he wishes to continue medication. Requests for sedatives, tranquillisers or antidepressants are common examples. An interesting aspect of repeat prescribing is the apparent increase in the number of prescriptions that are obtained via the receptionist [37, 38] and do not involve direct contact by the patient with the general practitioner. The majority [39] of repeat prescriptions represent routine request (81.8%), followed by sporadic treatments (10.4%) such as seasonal antihistamines and topical steroids. There is obviously a very large variation between different practices and although the attitude of the general practitioner is important, the attitude and action of the patient also makes a significant contribution. Balint and his colleagues [40] have examined the characteristics and the variants of the 'repeat prescription patient'. Recently [41] most concern has been expressed over the increase in psychoactive drugs — approximately 30% of all requests for repeat prescriptions.

These three examples illustrate positive or negative decision-making by patients with regard to treatments — either the decision not to self-medicate or seek professional care, or the decision to alter prescribed treatment. They demonstrate the degree to which medication is directly under the control of the patient and the significance and complexity of the decision-making process.

SAFETY

Although at present most attention is linked to the side-effects of prescribed drugs, it is useful to remember that some over-the-counter preparations can also have undesirable and indeed serious ill-effects.
serious ill-effects.

Pink disease [42, 43], erythroedema or acrodynia, as it was called, is an interesting example of a condition which was quite common in the 1930s but is now extinct. It was the result of chronic mercurial poisoning from teething powders which were freely available in chemists and grocery shops throughout the country. Currently, the possible serious side-effects of certain remedies used by some immigrant communities in Britain have been highlighted [44]. One remedy, bal-jivan chamcho, a general childrens remedy for diarrhoea, rickets and bronchitis, bears a striking similarity to the mercurial teething powders, but the metal involved is usually lead and originates from the spoon containing the child's medicine. Remedies used by Hakims and other practitioners of the Unani and Areyuvidic systems of medicine frequently contain a mixture of metallic substances, modern drugs and herbal remedies. Surma [45], used as a cosmetic and treatment for certain eye conditions, may contain lead, the dangers of which have been noted in children.

Two important recent reminders of possible serious side-effects of over-the-counter preparations are kidney damage from the analgesic, phenacetin, and the problem of subacute myelo-optic neuropathy (SMON) resulting from clioquinol (Enterovioform).

These few examples appear to be the exception rather than the rule, and from assessment by doctors [46] of the effectiveness and safety of self-medication, there is general agreement that it is safe, appropriate and unlikely to lead to delay in presenting to doctors the more serious problems. This last concern is most frequently voiced [47]. The risk of interaction [48] between self-medication, prescribed drugs and food or alcohol is a real but probably small problem.

As evidenced by recent public concern over thalidomide and whooping cough immunization, the problem of side-effects appears to be well-recognized and understood. However it is possible that there may be some changes in treating symptoms which represent the body's defence system, e.g. diarrhoea.

FAMILY, SOCIAL AND COMMUNITY INFLUENCES

In the process of definition, which is the first step in coping with a problematic health situation, as with other problems, an individual uses his 'stock of knowledge', which as Schutz and McHugh point out [49—51] is an accumulation of his own direct experiences, the knowledge of others' experiences, the influence of the media and professionals and complex community and social influences. After defining the problem, the choice of action is from a set of possible responses. Just as the individual's definition is the product of his life's history, of all his experiences, both social and individual, both direct and vicarious, through communication with others, so is his choice of 'recipes for action'.

If a symptom is defined as a trivial departure from normal, it may be ignored and left to vanish of its own accord. If trivial, but it interferes with function or is distressing or uncomfortable but recognized as part of a normally self-limiting illness, then symptomatic relief may be obtained from well-tried remedies, while normal recovery takes place. If the diagnosis is uncertain, the advice of family, friends, colleagues or a local expert may be sought. If it is more serious or persistent (either related to a recognized illness or the diagnosis is uncertain) there may be rapid recourse to a medical practitioner. Only a proportion of symptoms are even discussed within the family context and fewer still are referred to outside the family. This 'lay-referral system' as it has been termed [52], and the use of lay consultants is well-documented, and it varies according to the cultural environment and the social networks that exist in a particular community [53—55].

Pratt [56] has emphasized the central and continuing role of the family in the control of medication. He maintains that family interest and function 'require that they assert a degree of control over medication that permits them to assume full and timely servicing of members' health needs with minimum cost and bother, and protection of members from inappropriate and dangerous treatment by professionals'.

The inappropriateness of attempting to separate the various components of health care or neglecting the traditional, cultural, social and family influences is being increasingly recognized, and is one of the main tenets of the holistic approach to health [57].

THE PRESENT AND THE FUTURE

Clearly, at present, self-medication and other aspects of self-care form an enormous part of the overall activities related to promoting health, preventing illness and coping with symptoms and illness. A question that is often posed in Britain is why do people self-medicate when there is a freely available comprehensive National Health Service?

Self-medication is the traditional [58] way of coping with health problems and it is still normal to use it in situations which are defined as appropriate. There is clear evidence [59] of extensive community knowledge on health, illness and care, and by use of family and community resources most people seem to find little difficulty in deciding what conditions can be safely and appropriately treated without recourse to professional care [7]. In the opinion of those who consumed the medication [3], about two-thirds of all medicines taken by adults were said to be helpful. It is convenient in the case of trivial complaints to self-treat with remedies already in the household and not to have to seek professional care. There is a fear that patients may be seen as wasting the doctor's time; this may be related to a belief that the doctor will view the condition as trivial. Indeed this belief, and the complaints by general practitioners about wasting their time on trivial conditions, implies that patients should make more use of self-care. Alternatively, there may be a belief that professional care may be able to achieve nothing — in chronic conditions such as rheumatism, — or there may be a fear that the condition is fatal and here there may be anxiety about the repercussions of seeking professional care and the certainty of an adverse diagnoses. Dislike of doctors and previous bad experience with health professionals may also play a part. Closely linked to this is a dislike of bureaucracy and professionals and a desire by individuals to seek 'alternatives' which may be more under their control.

Self-medication may be a form of care on its own, or it may be a prelude to contact with a general practitioner or it may coexist [60]. It is estimated that approximately half of the patients attending for primary care had previously self-medicated. There is some conflicting evidence as to whether or not self-medication is a direct alternative to professional treatment. Dunnell and Cartwright [3] consider that in adults self-medication may be a direct alternative to professional care but in children self-treatment is apparently used to supplement professional consultation, although most other studies have not found evidence that it is a substitute to consulting the doctor. Blum [1] has suggested that the attitude towards medication is important and that persons with a greater drug experience and more experience of medical care, believed in the efficiency of medication and gave drugs to others as well as self-medicating, to a greater extent. Morell and Wale [7] consider that both self-medication and the propensity to consult are related to anxiety. Danaher and her colleagues [46, 60] suggest that those who attended general practitioners for a particular symptom tended to self-treat for an insufficient period of time before consultation, compared with non-attenders with the same symptom even though the severity of the symptom was similar. One factor which emerges repeatedly from studies [3, 7, 9, 12, 13, 15, 61] is that women dose themselves more than men. We can only speculate about the reasons [3] — perhaps it has to do with the feeling that women can less easily take to their beds than men, perhaps because they suffer from ailments more amenable to self-medication, perhaps because women do more shopping so over-the-counter preparations are more available to them, or perhaps they make greater use of social networks which are likely to advise and encourage various approaches to self-care.

Looking to the future, the present trends seem to be emphasizing an educational approach. It is perhaps a testimony to public commonsense and to the standards of the pharmaceutical companies that this sizeable section of the health care system appears relatively safe, acceptable and is not widely criticized. Much of the present information is based on studies examining particular aspects, sometimes involving small numbers and often using different methods and definitions. There is a need for further research, but the real challenge seems to be an educational one. Some call for general practitioners to take on new roles as health educators [62, 63]; Others [64, 65] have suggested that an enhanced role for the pharmacist would be a more logical focus for health education. It has been suggested that problems, policy and methods of education have for too long been directed by professionals and that groups in the community should assume responsibility for initiating and arranging this educational process — using the skills of professionals to meet the defined needs of the community. Many self-help groups have developed this approach as has the Women's Movement. An interesting example of a joint approach is the practice association [66] where patients and staff participate in deciding problems for discussion and educational sessions. This, and other examples of liaison with educational authorities, indicate the possibility of a health centre which might encompass a number of health promoting and health educational functions. Curriculum development [67] and the inclusion of many health topics in schools is another exciting area of innovation.

Home doctor books and medical encyclopaedias have a long-established place [58]. Recently there seems to have been a revival of interest and a number of new publications. Books such as *Take Care of Yourself. A consumer's Guide to Medical Care* [68] and *How to be Your Own Doctor* [69] sometimes contain comprehensive sections on diagnosis and self-treatment as well as advice on how to get the best out of health services. In contrast to the specific treatments recommended in such publications, a book such as *The Encyclopaedia of Alternative Medicine and Self-Help* [70], lists the many alternative approaches available, rather than promoting definite remedies. Finally there are books, such as *Medicines. A Guide for Everybody* [71], which sets out to provide information about drugs to people who have no medical training or knowledge, or a simpler booklet like the one issued by the Health Education Council on *Treating Yourself* [72].

CONCLUSION

Self-medication is a normal and appropriate part of the overall provision of health care. This is recognized by professionals who equally recognize that the general practitioner could not cope if self-care were to be abolished. New educational roles for professionals are suggested which in turn would involve change in curricula in professional education and training. New participation for patients is proposed which would result in an alteration in the traditional patient—professional relationship. There is a need to re-eximaine policy to see what resources are required to achieve these aims and to determine methods of evaluating any changes which are implemented.

Acknowledgement

The material for this paper is drawn from a review of self-care, entitled 'Participating in Health', which is currently being prepared by Dr J. McEwen, Dr C. J. M. Martini and Mrs N. Wilkins. The support of the Health Education Council in this work is gratefully acknowledged.

References

1. Blum, R. H. (1971). Normal drug use. In H.P. Dreitzel (ed.). *The Social Organisation of Health.* Recent Sociology No. 3 (London: Collier-Macmillan Ltd.)
2. Wadsworth, M. E. J., Butterfield, W. J. H. and Blaney R. (1971). *Health and Sickness: The choice of treatment* (London: Tavistock Publications).
3. Dunnell, K. and Cartwright, A. (1972). *Medicine Takers, Prescribers and Hoarders.* (London: Routledge and Kegan Paul).
4. Logan, W. P. D. and Brooke E. M. (1957). *The Survey of Sickness 1943 to 1952.* General Register Office Studies on Medical and Population Studies No. 12. (London: HMSO)
5. Kohn, R. and White, K. L. (eds) (1976). *Health Care: An International Study.* (London: Oxford University Press)
6. Pearse, I. H. and Crocker, L. H. (1943). *The Peckham Experiment.* (London: Allen and Unwin)
7. Morrell, D. C. and Wale, C. J. (1976). Symptoms perceived and recorded by patients. *J. R. Coll. Gen. Practit.,* **26**, 398
8. Brotherston, J. H. F. and Chave, S. P. W. (1956). General practice on a new housing estate. *Br. J. Prev. Soc. Med.,* **10**, 200
9. Martin, F. M., Brotherston, J. H. P. and Chave, S. P. W. (1957). Incidence of neurosis in a new housing estate. *Br. J. Prev. Soc. Med.,* **11**, 196
10. Ineichen, B. (1975). Neurotic wives in a modern residential suburb: a sociological profile. *Soc. Sci. Med.,* **9**, 481
11. Ineichen, B. and Hooper, D. (1974). Wives' mental health and children's behaviour problems in contrasting residential areas. *Soc. Sci. Med.,* **8**, 369
12. Bell, J. M. (1977). The use of general practitioner services by

young married women in a new town. B. Phil thesis, University of Dundee

13. Bell, J. M., Black, I., McEwen, J. and Pearson J. (1977). *Patterns of Illness. A Comparative Study in a New Town.* Report to Scottish Home and Health Dept.

14. Fanning, D. M. (1976). Families in flats. *Br. Med. J.,* **4**, 382

15. Banks, M. H., Beresford, S. A. R., Morrell, D. C., Waller, J. J. and Watkins, C. J. (1975). Factors influencing demand for primary medical care in women, aged 20—44 years. A preliminary report. *Int. J. Epidemiol.,* **4**, 189

16. Department of Health, Education and Welfare (1969) *Acute Conditions, Incidence and Associated Disability Series 10, No. 54.* US National Centre for Health Statistics (Washington)

17. Hinkle, L., Redmont, R., Plummer, N. and Wolff, H. G. (1960). An examination of the relation between symptoms, disability and serious illness, in two homogeneous groups of men and women. *Am. J. Public Health,* **50**, 1327

18. Alpert, J. J., Kosa, J. and Haggerty, R. J. (1967). A month of illness and health care among low-income families. *Public Health Rep.,* **82**, 705

19. Knapp, D. A. and Knapp, D. E. (1972). Decision making and self medication. *Am. J. Hosp. Pharm.,* **29**, 1004

20. Department of Health Education and Welfare (1969). *Chronic Conditions Causing Activity Limitation.* Series 10 No. 51. (Washington: U.S. National Center for Health Statistics)

21. Jefferys, M., Brotherston, J. H. F. and Cartwright, A. (1960). Consumption of medicines on a working-class housing estate. *Br. J. Prev. Soc. Med.,*

22. Fry, J. (1978). *A New Approach to Medicine. Principles and Priorities in Health Care.* (Lancaster: MTP Press)

23. Horder, J. and Horder, E. (1954). Illness in general practice. *Practitioner,* **173**, 177

24. Roney, J. G. and Nall, M. L. (1966). Medical practices in a community: an exploratory study - quoted in Pratt, L. (Ref. 56).

25. Leach, R. H. and White P. L. (1978). Use and wastage of prescribed medicines in the home. *J. R. Coll. Gen. Practit.* **28**, 32

26. Johnson and Johnson (1970). Medicine Chest Survey. Quoted in Pratt, L. (Ref. 56).

27. Hannay, D. R. (1975). A survey of symptoms and sickness behaviour in glasgow. Report to the Social Science Research Council (No. H.R. 1550).
28. Jones, R. V. H. (1976). Self-medication in a small community. *J. R. Coll. Gen. Practit.*, **26**, 410
29. Elliott-Binns, C. P. (1973). An analysis of lay medicine. *J. R. Coll. Gen. Practit.*, **23**, 255
30. Breckon, W. (1977). The Physick in the Herbs. *World Medicine*, **12**, 44
31. Food and Drug Administration (1972). A study of health practices and opinions. U.S. Department of Health, Education and Welfare
32. Roghmann, K. J. and Haggerty, R. J. (1972). The diary as a research instrument in the study of health and illness behaviour. *Med. Care*, **10**, 143
33. Hassinger, E. W. and McNemara, R. L. (1960). The families, their physicians, their health behavior in a northwest Missouri County. Quoted in Pratt, L. (Ref. 56).
34. Festinger, L. (1962). *A Theory of Cognitive Dissonance*. (London: Tavistock Publications)
35. Ley, P. (1974). Communication in the clinical setting. *B. J. Orthodont.*, **1**, 173
36. Stimson, G. V. (1974). Obeying doctor's orders: a view from the other side. *Soc. Sci. Med.*, **8**, 97
37. Madeley, J. (1974). Repeat prescribing via the receptionist in a group practice. *J. R. Coll. Gen. Practit.*, **24**, 425
38. Austin, R. and Parish, P. (1976), Prescriptions written by ancillary staff. *J. R. Coll. Gen. Practit.*, **26**, Supplement 44
39. Manasse, A. P. (1974). Repeat prescriptions in general practice. *J. R. Coll. Gen. Practit.*, **24**, 203
40. Balint, M., Hunt, J., Joyce, D., Marinker, M. and Woodcock, J. (1970). *Treatment or Diagnosis*. (London: Tavistock)
41. *J. R. Coll. Gen. Practit.* (1973). The medical use of psychotropic drugs,
42. Hart, F. D. (1978). Therapeutic poison pictures. *World Med.*,
43. Bodley Scott, Sir R. (ed.). (1978). *Price's Textbook of the Practice of Medicine, 12 ed.* p.271 (Oxford: University Press)
44. Davis, S. S. and Aslam, M. (1979). Health Care Needs of Asian Immigrants. Submitted for publication.
45. Ali, A. R., Smales, O. R. C. and Aslam, M. (1978). Surma and lead poisoning. *Br. Med. J.*, **2**, 915

46. Anderson, J. A. D., Buck, C., Danaher, K. and Fry, J. (1977). Users non-users of physicians. *J. R. Coll. Gen. Practit.,*
47. Goldsen, R. (1963). Patient delay in seeking cancer diagnosis: behavioural aspects. *J. Chronic Dis.,* 16, 427
48. Stockley, I. H. (1978). *Drug Interaction Alert, Aide Memoire on Interaction for Physicians and Pharmacists.* (Bracknell: Boehringer — Ingelheim).
49. Shutz, A. (1962). *Collected Papers I. The Problem of Social Reality.* Nathanson, M. (ed.). (The Hague: Martinus Nijhoff)
50. Schutz, A. (1964). *Collected Papers II. Studies in Social Theory.* Brodersen, A. (ed.). (The Hague: Martinus Nijhoff)
51. McHugh, P. (1968). *Defining the Situation: The Organization of Meaning in Social Interaction.* (Indianapolis: Bobbs-Merrill Co.)
52. Freidson, E. (1970). *The Profession of Medicine.* (New York: Dodd Mead and Co.)
53. Bott, E. (1971). *Family and Social Network. Rules Norms and External Relationships in Ordinary Urban Life.,* 2nd ed. (London: Tavistock)
54. Finlayson, A. (1974). Social networks as coping resources, lay help and consultation patterns used by women in husband's post-infarction careers. *Soc. Sci. Med.,* 10, 97
55. McKinaly, J. (1973). Social networks and utilization behaviour, *Soc. Forces,* 51, 275
56. Pratt, L. (1973). The significance of the family in medication. *J. Comp. Family Studies,* 4, 13
57. Editorial (1979). Holistic medicine. *N. Engl. J. Med.,* 1, 312
58. Woodward, J. and Richards, D. (1977). *Health Care and Popular Medicine in Nineteenth Century England.* (London: Croom Helm)
59. Office of Health Economics. (1968). *Without Prescription.* (London: OHF)
60. Williamson, J. D. and Danaher, K. (1978). *Self-care in Health.* (London: Croom Helm)
61. Lader, S. (1965). A Survey of the Incidence of Self-Medication. *Practitioner,* 194, 132
62. Donovan, C. F. (1977). A doctor's responsibility to his patients. *Proc. R. Soc. Med.,* 70, 21
63. Dingwall, D. (1975). *Patient Education in the Use of the National Health Service.* Paper Presented at a Conference on Patient Education in Primary Care, Dundee.
64. Sharpe, D. N. (1977). Role of the pharmacist in the community. A

pharmaceutiçal role. *Pharm. J.*, **219**, 280
65. Webb, B. (1976). The retail pharmacist and drug treatment. *J. R. Coll. Gen. Practit.*, **26**, Supplement 81
66. Wilson, A. T. M. (1977). Patient participation in a primary care unit. *Br. Med. J.*, **1**, 398
67. Department of Education and Science (1978). *Curriculum Development. 11—16. Health Education in the Secondary School Curriculum.* Working papers by Health Education Committee of H.M. Inspectorate.
68. Vickery, D. M. and Freis, J. F. (1976). *Take Care of Yourself. A Consumer's Guide to Medical Care.* (Reading, Mass.: Addison-Wesley Pub. Co.)
69. Sehnert, K. W. (1975). *How to be Your Own Doctor — Sometimes.* (New York. Grosset and Dunlap)
70. Hulke, M. (ed.) (1978). *The Encyclopaedia of Alternative Medicine and Self Help.* (London: Rider and Company)
71. Parish, P. (1976). *Medicines. A Guide for Everybody.* (Harmondsworth: Penguin)
72. Health Education Council (1974). *Treating Yourself — A Guide to Self Medication.* (London: HEC)

8

Concluding commentary

J. A. D. ANDERSON

INTRODUCTION

In relation to the first aim of this Workshop it would appear that consensus exists among the participants, who are drawn from a wide range of academic, practising and marketing disciplines. This is in spite of the fact that no-one who attended appears to have been unduly inhibited from expressing an opinion, which, in turn, could mean that only those likely to concur have been asked to attend. This, however, seems unlikely as notices inviting participation were sent to all medical schools in Great Britain and Ireland as well as to a wide range of organizations and individuals associated with several medical specialists including general practice, various sections of the nursing profession including health visiting, and hospital and community pharmacists, there have also been contributions by participants from the Consumers' Association and an Area Health Authority.

There is general agreement that self-medication is not only practised widely but is here to stay. It is part of the self-caring process which occurs even under the sort of conditions in which comprehensive health and social services are provided with little or no charge to those who judge themselves to be in need; indeed some form of self-medication is necessary under such circumstances if the statutory services are not to be overwhelmed by unlimited demands.

On the other hand some of the pigeons, in the form of hypotheses implicit in the questions posed by the introductory papers, have come home to roost in the comments of the rapporteurs and the discussions which they have provoked. Major problems of precise identification remain and have been raised repeatedly in discussion both in the working groups and in plenary session. These can be expressed as four pairs of contrasting statements:

(1) Self-reliance is worth the risk of occasional catastrophe in the use of home medicines; or, legislation must protect the public against every possible misuse and potential danger in relation to any commodity freely available.

(2) Community pharmacists are health educators and diagnosticians, and as such should be encouraged to undertake the role of apothecaries; or, those making profit from wholesale or retail sale of medicines cannot be expected to give advice on self-medication without bias.

(3) Any medication should be available for sale to the public providing specific indications on dose restrictions are clearly stated and no attempt at polypharmacy is permitted; or, only homeopathic doses should be used in home medicines so that wide permutations may be combined safely in a single polyvalent remedy.

(4) Only those certified as competent to treat illness should be allowed to make decisions about the use of medicaments; or all possible steps should be taken to reduce the load on the National Health Service in general and on family practitioners in particular.

As with any contrasting extremes of opinion the best solution is seldom if ever found at one end of the spectrum but rather within a central grey zone which extends over quite a broad band and which has blurred margins. It is perhaps noteworthy in this connection that views have been expressed forcefully from those representing the many factions involved in this multi-disciplinary Workshop; on the other hand there has been little evidence of frank polarization, and it is on this basis that the conclusion about consensus would appear to be justified.

ANSWERING THE QUESTIONS

Some of the questions posed by the authors of the precirculated papers (Chapters 3 to 6) and also those agreed among the participants at the preliminary plenary session were clearly easier to answer than others.

Generalizations are dangerous; however it would appear that the questions considered by Groups A and C (Chapters 3 and 5) which which tended to be concerned with the products themselves, their distribution and use permitted more straightforward answers than the questions facing Groups B and D (Chapters 4 and 6) in which concepts and relationship problems were considered. Among the exceptions to such a generalization might be mentioned the attitudes of the elderly to the prolonged use of home medicines which was considered by Group A (Chapter 3); another exception, considered by Group B (Chapter 4), is the identification of symptom complexes which could be expected to respond to specific home medicines.

Even when it was not possible to give firm answers to the questions which had been posed, the action suggested to redeem the situation was more clearcut in relation to some topics than others. Accordingly, it could be tempting to tackle those problems which appear to admit of a simple solution even though it does not necessarily follow that easy answers will be found. Indeed there appear to be many areas of possible research suggested by the groups that could provide useful information fairly quickly for those concerned with caring for the public, health education and the manufacture and marketing of home remedies.

However, nettles must also be grasped and the debate about the place of home medicines in a comprehensive system of state care is unlikely to be resolved until an answer is found to such complex proposals as that put forward by Group B (Chapter 4): that population subgroups likely to be benefited and those likely to be disadvantaged must first be identified and then educated as to how best to meet their respective needs. Also difficult to achieve, but undoubtedly very important in the field of self-medication, are the interprofessional boundaries and the capacity of different professional groups to educate each other across these boundaries, which formed a substantial part of the deliberations of Group D (Chapter 6) — even though the question of how to educate the educators had not been posed explicitly. A quick solution is unlikely and indeed there may be no solution but some attempt must be made to resolve the tendency to isolationism among professional groups; then and only then is it likely that these groups can combine satisfactorily to educate the public at large on this or any other health issue of importance. The same level of complexity applies in finding solutions through research and experiment to many of the other problems arising from the discussions at this Workshop.

RESEARCH RECOMMENDATIONS

The recommendations and opinions of the four discussion groups have been presented by the rapporteurs (Chapters 3 to 6) and it would be superfluous to repeat them in full. However, it is perhaps useful to draw some of the threads together.

Broadly speaking there are requirements for two types of research: fact-finding surveys are needed to acquire reliable information, and experiments must be launched to test hypotheses. Many of the proposals appear to fall fairly clearly into one or other of these categories; thus the following are examples of suggested studies seeking to collate or clarify information:

(A) What are the extent and circumstances under which long-term home medication is carried out among the elderly?

(B) What are the perceptions of effectiveness held by the users of home medicines?

(C) What evidence is there of drug misuse among those seeking medical advice for backache?

(D) How deficient is the knowledge of patients about medicines and their appropriate and safe use?

By way of contrast the following are hypotheses which seem to require some form of experimental design:

(A) Multiple-ingredient home medicines are no more effective than single-ingredient preparations yet they carry a greater potential for unwanted effects.

(B) Medicines for specified common symptom complexes require explicit user guidelines.

(C) The 'expectation effect' makes a contribution beyond the pharmacological action of a home medication because of the impact of advertising.

(D) A community pharmacist attached to a primary care team makes a greater contribution than one practising from his own premises.

Neither list exhausts the suggestions of any of the groups but consideration of the four reports could result in many of the proposals (either in whole or in part) being allocated under one or other of these two headings. However, it is either inherent in a few suggestions listed by the rapporteurs or it has emerged in the course of the discussions which followed each Group report that the requirement to collect and collate

*recommendations of Group A (Chapter III), Group B (Chapter IV) etc.

further information forms an essential and integral prerequisite of some definite experiment. Suggestions under this heading include:

(A) To what extent are home medicines used on a long-term basis by the elderly? Limitations on the duration of use should be considered if a real problem is identified by this investigation.

(B) What opportunities exist for educating health personnel and the lay public? Such opportunities if properly used will improve the quality of self-medication.

(C) What sort of information and advice is given by community pharmacists in relation to home medicines? Extended training of pharmacists will improve the quality of this service.

(D) To what extent do patients feel dissatisfied with medicines prescribed by health service agencies and for what complaints? Improved treatment of complaints identified in this way will reduce the misuse of home medicines.

Other proposals which appear at first sight to be merely seeking further information or clarification may well result in exposing problems which require experiments for their resolution. By definition it is impossible to identify precisely what the subsequent experiment might be; however, it would not be difficult to imagine experiments developing from the answers to such questions as:

(A) How do the public equate the financial cost of home medication with the delays and inconvenience of using health services?

(B) What are the deficiences in existing methods and styles of traditional medical practice as seen by the public?

(C) Is the information in relation to home medicines which is expected by the public compatible with that recommended by doctors and/or pharmacists?

(D) What information does the individual seeking relief from symptoms require about the disorders themselves before starting to self-medicate?

Furthermore, some of the suggestions for experiments may well require information to be collected before the experiment can be properly planned. Hypotheses which might possibly occur in this category when they are considered more closely include:

(A) The placebo effect of a home medicine demonstrated in a

117

controlled clinical situation is applicable to the self-caring situation.

(B) Self-care is a potent change agent in educating both health personnel and the lay public about health care problems.

(C) There are measurable side effects among those indulging in 'secondary home-medication' for routine relief of specified chronic conditions.

(D) A properly developed triage system for the public assists in deciding when not to treat without medical advice.

FURTHER WORKSHOPS AND DISCUSSIONS

Finally there are suggestions for further study in fields parallel or related to self-medication which would seem to require the convening of complementary workshops in order to crystallize thinking and give more detailed consideration to what further research is required. Indeed in the open discussions following the reports from the groups the need for some of these workshops was stated explicitly by more than one participant. Topics might include:

(1) Safe and effective storage of home medicines including child resistant packaging and 'medicine cupboard life'.

(2) The responsibilities of statutory and voluntary funding bodies in relation to a topic such as self-medication which does not appear to fall within the remit of a single organisation.

(C) Extension of the open purchase principle to some 'scheduled' medicines and the safeguards (for example only in the presence of a qualified pharmacist) that would be necessary.

(D) The alternatives to medicinal treatment and the broader issues of self-care.

It would be invidious for any individual to allocate priorities to the list of proposals not least because research programmes must be based on a combination of interests. Thus there may be several factions seeking answers to the same questions. There are also some research projects which are much more attractive than others to those who have to carry them out. Furthermore some projects must be based on those academic departments which have appropriate expertise and research capability to obtain and interpret the information on the one hand and to develop and test hypotheses on the other. These depend to a large extent on the disciplines of departmental members and their prime interests be that pharmacology, health education, community medicine or any of the numerous other specialists represented at this conference.

FOLLOW-UP MEETING

In order to draw up a list of priorities on a reasonably broad base a follow-up meeting was convened to which the authors of the papers and the four rapporteurs were invited to attend. As predicted priorities varied with the interests and discipline of the participants but the following is a consensus view of these priorities:

(a) Study Group A — Use and Misuse of Home Medicines

Suggested Project	*Suggested Priority*
1. Effect of cost in limiting self-medication — — particularly among old-age pensioners.	4
2. Controlled trial of home medicines and placebos.	4
3. Interaction of different elements in multi-ingredient preparations.	5
4. Interaction between ingredients of home medicines and prescribed medicines (including the knowledge or lack of knowledge that practitioners have about which medicaments are being used by their patients).	5
5. "Illicit" use of home medicines (with and without prescribed medicines such as barbiturates) in acute and chronic situations.	1
6. Effect of home medicines in causing drowsiness	3
7. Effect of home medicines on early pregnancy.	1
8. Extent to which home medicines are retained "on the shelf" in contrast to prescribed medicines in campaigns for handling in unwanted medicaments.	2

(b) Study Group B — Communication, Advertising and Education

Suggested Project	*Suggested Priority*
1. Extent to which self-medication is used by patients because of unsatisfactory experience with health services.	2/3

2. Relationship between self-medication and health education of both health personnel and the public.	2/3
3. Expectation effect of self-medication in different groups of the population (age, sex, social class).	1
4. Use of self-medication in chronic episodes.	1
5. Development of user guide-lines for self-medication of common sympton complexes.	3

(c) Study Group C — Products' Suitability for Home Care

Suggested Project	*Suggested Priority*
1. Harmful effects of "secondary" home medication in spasmodic use.	1
2. Expectation effect in symptomatic home medication.	2
3. Role of the community pharmacist in advising new users of home medication.	2
4. Advising those using home medications chronically on the change in use.	2
5. Methods of advising the public on the interaction between home medicines and secondary home medication.	2
6. What information should be given to the public by community pharmacists?	2
7. What information should be given to the public on the pack?	3
8. Defining channels of communcation between health service workers in general and the public.	2
9. Role of health visitors and other nurses in the primary care team in giving advice on self-medication.	1
10. Use of symbols or diagrams in addition to written instructions on labels.	2
11. What additional symptoms might be suitable for primary home medication (including the extension of the range of substances available for open purchase)?	2

(d) Study Group D — Relations with Health Care Professions and Public

Suggested Project	Suggested Priority
1. Development of a try-out system of when and when not to treat without medical advice.	1
2. Role of a pharmacist as a member of the primary care team in health centres.	2
3. The use of drug information centres for lay enquiries.	3

Index